CHANGE OF HEART

CHANGE OF HEART

The Bodhisattva Peace Training of Chagdud Tulku

REVISED EDITION

∾

Compiled and Edited by
LAMA SHENPEN DROLMA

Iron Knot Press

Printed in the United States of America

Title: Change of Heart: the Bodhisattva Peace Training of Chagdud Tulku /
Lama Shenpen Drolma.
Published by Padma Publishing, 2013

Description: Revised Edition / Iron Knot Press, 2022.
Identifiers: EISBN 978-1-7362878-3-5 / Paperback ISBN
978-1-7362878-2-8

Iron Knot Press
PO Box 3094
Silver City, NM 88062-3094
Email: info@ironknotpress.org /website: www.ironknotinstitute.org

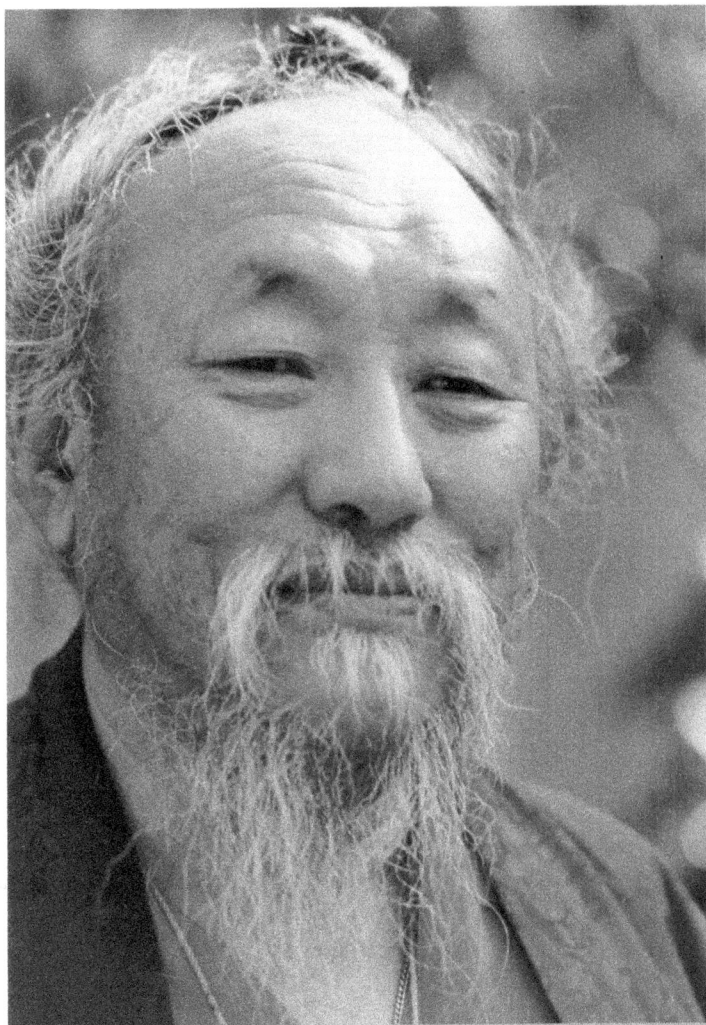

Dedicated to the fulfillment of the enlightened intent of
HIS EMINENCE CHAGDUD TULKU RINPOCHE

Contents

List of Meditations

Editor's Preface

THIS BOOK IS FOR THOSE who want to change—their hearts, their minds, the world. It is a guide, a manual of simple, accessible, and quietly revolutionary steps that individuals can take to transform their lives and the lives of others. On whatever level the teachings presented here are applied—from the intimate sphere of personal experience, to the complex dynamics of family, community, national, and even international relations—they will lead infallibly toward fulfillment and peace.

These teachings are drawn from a series of trainings conducted by His Eminence Chagdud Tulku Rinpoche, my teacher, respectfully and affectionately known simply as "Rinpoche" (Precious One) by all who knew him. He embodied and demonstrated the heart of the sacred dharma—the Buddhist teachings—and his realization of their inner meaning was so profound that he could convey their essence to all kinds of people, regardless of their life circumstances. I think it is safe to say that no one who met him remained untouched by his qualities of unfathomable wisdom and compassion.

Born in 1930 in eastern Tibet, Rinpoche studied with some of the greatest lamas of the twentieth century. He undertook extensive scholastic and meditative training, including two traditional three-year retreats. In 1959, during the consolidation of power by the Communist Chinese, he fled Tibet. For the next twenty years, he helped develop several Tibetan refugee communities in India and Nepal, serving the residents as lama and physician.

In 1979 he came to the United States, where he established Chagdud Gonpa Foundation, named after his monastery in eastern Tibet. Over the years, he created numerous centers for the study and practice of Vajrayana Buddhism throughout North and South America, Europe, and Australia. In 1996 Rinpoche moved to Brazil, where the vast range of his activity continued to grow. He taught tirelessly through the very evening of his passing in November 2002.

I met Rinpoche in the course of a search for spiritual tools that would help to overcome limitations of my heart and mind that had grown increasingly apparent as I attempted to respond to suffering in the world around me. My effectiveness had been gradually undermined by periodic discouragement and disappointment—a problem common to many working on behalf of others, whether on a personal or public level.

In Rinpoche's transmission of the 2,500-year-old tradition of Buddhism, I was surprised and profoundly grateful to find the very practical, accessible wisdom I had been looking for, as well as methods for navigating my modern American life. As a foundation for kindness and as a preparation for helping others, the teachings were life-altering. Moved by their extraordinary effectiveness, I was also concerned that they reach those who might be uncomfortable receiving them in a Buddhist context.

In his inimitable style, in order to benefit as many beings as possible, Rinpoche created an innovative format for presenting these tools—the essential methods of Mahayana Buddhism offered in such a way that anyone of any faith, political or philosophical persuasion could use them. And so the Bodhisattva Peace Training was born.

In the last fourteen years of his life, Rinpoche gave the Bodhisattva Peace Training to hundreds of individuals in a multitude of settings. I had the privilege of participating in a number of these trainings, both as student and as interpreter of his unique English. There are truly no words to describe the experience of sitting with him among people of all ages, backgrounds, and spiritual paths as their minds opened. Whether they were coming from places of deep rage, depression, confusion, or strong political or social ideologies, Rinpoche gently, persistently, and unfailingly showed them the loving, kind, and compassionate depths of their hearts.

In 1996 I began the process of bringing the Bodhisattva Peace Training into book form, sorting through transcripts of trainings Rinpoche had conducted with a variety of participants from diverse backgrounds. Work on the book intensified after Rinpoche's visits to Iron Knot Ranch, his center in southern New Mexico, where I had served as resident lama since 1999. A number of us at the ranch had aspired for some time to fulfill Rinpoche's long-held wish that these teachings become more widely available through the establishment of an institute where sincere practitioners could train and become qualified to teach the methods of the Bodhisattva Peace Training. During these visits, Rinpoche described his vision of the development of such an institute at Iron Knot Ranch and emphasized the importance of completing this book.

Finally, in the summer and fall of 2002, I went into retreat to finish the manuscript. That November, on my way to Brazil to read him the most recent draft, I received the news that he was experiencing severe chest pains. The next night he died.

So it is with deep sadness and regret that I complete this book without his feedback and corrections. I have tried to the best of my ability to preserve both the tone and content of his transmission of these teachings, and I take full responsibility for any errors or misrepresentations.

I have attempted here to convey the spirit of a Bodhisattva Peace Training with an intimate gathering of students. This necessarily involves the repetition of certain themes, which naturally takes place in such a setting. Most chapters begin with a teaching followed by questions and answers. A majority of the questions were pulled from transcripts and are articulated by eleven fictitious characters whose backgrounds and concerns mirror the array of Bodhisattva Peace Training students. Many chapters in the first two sections close with suggested formal meditation practices. Although Rinpoche taught these meditations in various ways over the years, in this book they follow a format that many participants have found helpful in trainings I have conducted since Rinpoche authorized me to give these teachings.

When we put the teachings into practice, change happens in the mind. Through our reading, questioning, and engagement, they come alive as direct personal experience. Rather than presenting spiritual truths theoretically, this book reflects Rinpoche's insistence that the genuine spiritual path involves constant practice throughout one's life. When diligently applied, these methods serve as stepping-stones to an awakening of compassion—an inexhaustible source of strength and resolve—from which change can be skillfully effected, both inwardly and outwardly.

Although these teachings are offered in a far more secular and casual manner than is traditional in Buddhist settings, non-Buddhist readers may nonetheless find themselves challenged by certain principles, such as reincarnation and the existence of other realms of reality. Whether these are taken literally or metaphorically, the wisdom of the teachings becomes self-evident when the methods Rinpoche shares are applied to the reader's own mind.

Those who had the great fortune to sit in Rinpoche's presence know that his spoken words were imbued with a wordless transmission that illuminated the heart. I pray that after a long, loving, but nonetheless human editorial process, the radiance of his wisdom still shines through.

Through the power of Rinpoche's blessings and those of all enlightened guides, may this work make possible for all beings an awakening to the limitless wisdom and compassion that is their true nature.

Lama Shenpen Drolma
Iron Knot Ranch, New Mexico, USA
2003

Preface to the Revised Edition

DURING HIS LIFETIME, His Eminence Chagdud Tulku Rinpoche created vast benefit throughout the world. He demonstrated the unceasing activity of a bodhisattva—one who is committed to alleviating the suffering of others while simultaneously establishing their enduring well-being. That he taught extensively concerning how we could do the same, bringing his depth of wisdom and compassion to the everyday dilemmas we all face, is a cause for great rejoicing.

Through the teachings found in this book, we can begin to experience the embrace of wisdom and sanity that comes from giving rise to awakened mind, the very heart of the bodhisattva. Truly the remedy for all that ails this world, it can be nurtured and expressed by anyone, regardless of religion, nationality, race, gender, income, health, or age. Of the vast array of thoughts and experience the human mind can give rise to, there is nothing more transformative than the simple profundity of a genuinely kind and good heart.

Many of the principles articulated here are relatively easy to comprehend and common to a variety of spiritual traditions. However, the actual experience of awakened mind takes place beyond the confines of any teaching, and ultimately beyond the realm of conceptual thought. Leading us skillfully to this awakened mind, Chagdud Tulku guides us through a time-honored instruction made accessible to our contemporary lives through the Bodhisattva Peace Training.

This practice involves three essential steps. First, we encounter teachings from a qualified lama or instructor. Then, we deeply contemplate what we have read or heard in order to determine its validity and relevance. We ask questions, identify doubts, and resolve confusion and misunderstanding. Finally, we meditate, blending the teachings with our mind and heart until we become one with them.

Being honest with ourselves about what's actually arising under the surface of our mind and heart at any given moment, and genuinely transforming anything other than good heart, takes years of experience. Stabilizing, deepening, and expanding that kind heart into a seamless experience of the awakened mind is ultimately a lifelong practice. What matters is not how long it takes, but that it happens authentically, for it is the accumulation of choices we make, moment by moment, that determines our future experience.

In our contemporary world of instantaneous access to knowledge, immediate gratification, and instant pain relief, we are accustomed to quick fixes. It would therefore be understandable to think that simply through reading, we could be changed permanently by a book like this and carry its meaning consistently into our daily lives.

But reading is only the first step in a lifelong journey. If we don't thoroughly engage the training, the values we hold so dear can be swept away by the tsunamis of our daily existence. We have spent a lifetime developing responses to pain and difficulty. Changing these old habits is like trying to reverse the momentum of a boulder tumbling down a mountainside. It requires great effort, skill, patience, perseverance, and no small amount of courage. But as we move closer to the realization that life's meaning and purpose can be found in benefiting others, the strength and sincerity of our efforts will be reflected in the world around us. Through this process that is at once tender and profound, a metamorphosis occurs that fundamentally alters our understanding of ourselves, of others, and of reality itself.

If you feel a resonance with Rinpoche's words—a yearning, even, to make your life and heart one with their meaning—spend time contemplating them, deeply, as they apply to life as you've known it. Then meditate on them, again, and again, when alone and in the world, throughout the day, every day, until their essence arises spontaneously as lived experience. Only when we genuinely live these teachings can our lives and our work in the world be transformed. Like gently washing away the impurities obscuring a luminous gem, we will slowly discover the treasury of our inherent positive qualities.

I am confident that whatever effort you put into this exploration will prove meaningful both to you and to those around you as you share your inspiration, not through words but through example, in the reflection in the world around you of the loving kindness in your heart.

It was Rinpoche's aspiration that the teachings contained in the Bodhisattva Peace Training would radiate out into the world, from one awakened heart to another. For this reason, he conceived of a program that would nourish the deepening practice of the awakened mind for all interested students, and also serve to certify as trainers those committed to the extensive preparation that is necessary. This training is now unfolding through the development of sister institutes in North and South America. When undertaken sincerely and diligently, this training offers the opportunity for genuine cultivation of the awakened mind under the direction and guidance of an authorized teacher, with support from others undergoing the same process. Rinpoche's wish was that this program would capture the authenticity, depth, and continuity of the training that he received from his teachers who, in turn, received it from their teachers, in an unbroken lineage dating back to the words of the Buddha himself.

These proven methods for awakening the mind and heart have been applied over the centuries, generation after generation, demonstrating their efficacy and power to transform our shared human experience. Meant to be practiced as a whole, each aspect of this extensive training supplements, empowers, and clarifies the next. Through this process, one is changed. And having begun to awaken one's own inherent positive qualities, one can help others to do the same, regardless of manifold life experiences.

I pray that the revised edition of this book with its expanded meditation instructions enriches the lives of all who make connection with it. May we take Chagdud Tulku's teachings to heart, and bring about temporary and ultimate benefit for all living beings.

Lama Shenpen Drolma
Iron Knot Ranch, New Mexico, USA
October 2014

Acknowledgments

WITHOUT THE INCOMPARABLE KINDNESS of His Eminence Chagdud Tulku Rinpoche, who made the West his home, thousands of sincere students would never have had the opportunity to receive authentic transmission of the exalted Vajrayana Buddhist teachings, to experience the heart of the Mahayana path through the lively format of the Bodhisattva Peace Training, or to benefit from the vast wisdom and compassion found in his books. Thank you, Rinpoche.

Deepest gratitude goes to my family and to Chagdud Khadro and Lama Drimed Norbu for their help as this project came to fruition; to Rinpoche's other interpreters during these trainings, Chagdud Khadro and Lama Tsering Everest; to Jane Barnes, Michael Bradfute, Casey McGee, Kimberley Snow, Barry Spacks, and, especially, Lama Tsultrim Palmo for their editorial contributions; to Linda Pinkham for her diligent inputting; to Linda Baer, Gina Phelan, Anna Smith, and Dan Tesser of Padma Publishing and others of the Chagdud Gonpa and Chagdud Lhundrub Ling sanghas who helped in many ways; and last, but not least, to Kim McLaughlin and a generous sponsor for everything they have done to make it possible for this book to come out at this time.

PART I

A Change of Heart

1

The Bodhisattva Peace Training

FROM THE TIME that I was a small child growing up in eastern Tibet, my kind teachers impressed upon me that the essential point of life is to develop the positive qualities inherent in the mind and to use them to help others. We may feel educated and capable if we have spent many years in school, in a trade, profession, or the arts, but most likely have not been formally trained in loving kindness or learned the true causes of peace and contentment.

This book presents just such a course of instruction, called the Bodhisattva Peace Training. Although "bodhisattva" is a Buddhist word, this training is not just for Buddhists. It offers methods that anyone of any faith can use to enhance mind's positive qualities, the source of benefit for ourselves and others, while reducing self-centered and negative habits, the source of harm for ourselves and others.

Such training is crucial if we aspire to have a positive impact—whether in a troubled relationship, family, workplace, community, or world. Our current perilous state of affairs has arisen from the conviction that each of us, regardless of our self-identity—as Christians, Buddhists, whites, blacks, Westerners, Easterners—knows the only way to true happiness. Most of us have never seriously considered that we might be wrong. We try to change or correct others, to convert them to our own way of seeing, then think we are clever if we succeed in doing so.

The truth is that we can rarely force others to act as we think they should or deter them from doing things we don't like. No matter how much we may want them to, it is unlikely that they will act according to our wishes, and we can seldom prevent difficulties from arising. We need to realize that our habitual approach to challenges—trying to change everything and everyone else—is ineffective. It fails to address the root of the problem, which is the negativity within our own mind.

Trying to change the world without changing our mind is like trying to clean the dirty face we see in the mirror by scrubbing the glass. However vigorously we clean it, our reflection will not improve. Only by washing our own face and combing our own unkempt hair can we alter the image. Similarly, if we want to help create conditions that foster peace and well-being in the world, we first need to reflect these qualities ourselves.

According to an old Buddhist saying, the world is like a great field filled with thorns and sharp objects; rather than trying to cover it with leather, it is far easier to wear a pair of leather shoes. We face a host of thorny issues with unlimited potential for dissent, strife, and bloody conflict. None of us, not even the most powerful leader, can remedy them all.

If we are to fulfill the short-term goal of resolving conflict, and the ultimate goal of eliminating all our flaws and making evident our positive qualities, we must rely on spiritual methods. Intellectual understanding alone will not make possible the profound inner peace that can influence others. Like mending a hole in our pants by sewing on a patch, we must use the methods of the spiritual path to stitch our understanding to the fabric of our being. We begin with the sincere wish to benefit others as much as ourselves. Recognizing that they want to be free of suffering and find happiness as much as we do, we seek ways of caring equally and simultaneously for ourselves and others. Over time, we expand the scope of our motivation, increasingly placing others' needs before our own. We cultivate boundless, unbiased compassion—not just for our children, friends, parents, or associates, but for all beings alike, without preference.

Such compassion—the desire to alleviate the suffering of all beings equally—is part of the meaning of the Sanskrit term "bodhisattva." *Bodhi* refers to wisdom mind, which is completely selfless. *Sattva* can be translated as "hero." A bodhisattva is someone who has taken on the sole task of meeting the needs of others, no matter how difficult that might be. His self-centeredness has been reduced to the point where wisdom, love, and compassion arise naturally, benefiting any situation. Motivated only by concern for others, he would offer his own life without regret if he saw that it would be of help. So the mind of the bodhisattva is heroic, vast, and of limitless benefit.

We cannot say that we are true bodhisattvas when we first give rise to the altruistic wish to serve others, but that is where we start. We then strive to develop selflessness in every aspect of our lives and to eliminate everything obscuring our natural positive qualities. The end result—what we call enlightenment in the Buddhist tradition—is the ability to help anyone who sees, hears, touches, or remembers us. Such benefit is spontaneous, unceasing, and unimpeded.

The Bodhisattva Peace Training begins where we are, as people who wish to develop greater compassion and love for those close to us. Then we practice extending compassion and love again and again, until our limitations and obstacles fall away and our inherent qualities increase immeasurably in scope and impact. This is the transformative purpose of the training—to introduce methods for reducing our self-centered, negative, and harmful thoughts, words, and actions and increasing positive and beneficial ones.

The training spans three to five days. A topic is presented and participants ask questions, reflect and meditate on it, then share how the teachings relate to their own experience and how their thinking has been affected by what they have learned. Contemplating and discussing the teachings in this way makes it easier to integrate them into daily life.

For the spiritual power of peace to touch every person on this earth, it must radiate out from a profound peace within our own mind: across political and religious barriers, and across the barriers of ego and self-righteousness. To this end, we should seek an inner peace so pure and stable that we cannot be moved to anger by violence or to selfish attachment and fear by those who view or confront us with contempt and hatred. We can achieve such stability only by purifying mind's poisons—ignorance, anger, attachment, jealousy, and pride; then we can clearly see that war and suffering are but their outer reflections. The essential difference between true peacemakers and those who wage war of any sort is the presence of extraordinary patience and discipline in the minds of the peacemakers as they work with these pervasive poisons. If we truly understand this, we will never allow ourselves to be defeated from within or without.

In Tibetan Buddhism, the peacock symbolizes the bodhi-sattva. A peacock is said to eat poisonous plants, transforming their toxins into the radiant colors of its feathers. It does not poison itself. In the same way, we who advocate peace must not poison ourselves with anger but regard with equanimity those who perpetrate violence, remaining constantly aware of our own state of mind. If we become angry in our efforts, we must pull back and regain our compassionate perspective. Without anger, perhaps we will penetrate the terrible delusion that gives rise to violence and hellish suffering.

From the clear space of our own inner peace, our compassion can expand to include all those caught in the tragic web of rage—aggressors and victims alike. True compassion is aroused by suffering of any sort, the suffering of every being. It is not tied to right or wrong, attachment or aversion. The work of peace is thus a spiritual path in itself, a means to develop the perfect qualities of mind that can be brought to bear in extreme suffering, urgent necessity, and death.

Substantial change happens slowly, and, in the midst of crisis, more slowly still. By starting with our own mind and working outward, we can affect others in extraordinary ways. A candle can bring a measure of light into the darkest room; a bright electric light will banish the darkness completely. The bodhisattva's powerful ability to benefit others is like that electric light; our current ability to help, more like the candle. Even so, one candle can light another, which can light the next, and so on until darkness fades. In this way, may the lamp of these teachings illuminate the minds of beings until the whole world blazes with light.

2

Pure Motivation

WE ASPIRE THROUGH this training to bring peace and benefit to our lives and to the world. The purer our motivation for receiving these teachings, the greater our ability to create benefit as we integrate them into our hearts and activities. Acting out of self-interest, attachment, and aversion is like cooking with a filthy pot. No matter how appealing the ingredients, or how long and carefully we cook them, the pot will only spoil the food.

Self-interest severely limits our ability to help. Self-clinging establishes a boundary between ourselves—including all we take to be ours—and everything else. We tend to isolate what we believe, need, and want for ourselves from the beliefs, needs, and desires of others. Such attachment leads to fixation on our own ideas, family, community, or country. We exaggerate the value of whatever we call "mine," imagining ourselves and "ours" to be uniquely important. This perspective separates, binds, and restricts us, making openness impossible. We react with aversion to not getting what we want, as well as to getting what we do not want. Attachment and aversion are like a twin-headed demon; they are two sides of the same coin.

Although we may aspire to help, we often find ourselves hampered by negativity and mental habits that perpetuate suffering and conflict rather than create happiness and harmony. Our intention to aid someone we sympathize with might be compromised by aversion toward someone who has injured her or by our desire to gain or achieve something through our actions. If in our efforts to help we become judgmental and self-righteous, if we angrily try to control or retaliate against someone, then our intention is tainted by pride and aversion. If our motivation for helping others is marred by desire, anger, or self-interest, we are like a doctor who administers sweet-tasting medicine laced with poison. It might seem delicious in the short run, but will ultimately only cause harm.

The mind is like a fertile field. If we contaminate it with the poisons of ignorance, desire, anger, jealousy, and pride, we will inevitably produce poisonous crops. Acting carelessly or harmfully toward others, or working for our own benefit at the expense of others, will only create limitation and suffering. Medicinal seeds—wholesome, virtuous acts of kindness, love, and compassion—will produce the fruits of peace and benefit. Actions that are both positive and negative will produce a mixture of happiness and sadness. This is the principle of karma. Karma originates in the mind. Our thoughts give rise to words and actions, and these have consequences. We cannot plant poisonous seeds and expect edible or medicinal fruit. When we begin to see the negative results of our self-centeredness, we understand why we must carefully choose which seeds to plant. Our future is in our own hands.

If our motivation is truly to help everyone, we must reduce our own negativity and learn to develop equal love and compassion for all beings. This means that we must try to help both victim and aggressor. In the case of a murder that is about to take place, our impulse is to defend the victim, but ideally we would also act out of compassion for the aggressor, to try to protect him from the consequences of killing. If he follows his murderous impulse, he will soon be estranged from everyone he has ever known or loved. He will ruin his life and destroy his chances for happiness. Thinking only of the short term, he has no idea what could be in store for him, a degree of suffering that we wouldn't wish on anyone. So as difficult as it seems, we must cultivate the same compassion for him as for the victim. One is suffering now; the other will suffer in the future. Equal compassion is truly great compassion.

Similarly, in the arena of world peace, we all wish to protect those ravaged by war, yet those who wage war will eventually experience the negative consequences of their actions. Because of the aggressors' power and arrogance, and the terrible suffering they inflict, it may be very hard for us to feel compassion for them. Nonetheless, we need to hold war-makers and victims in the same compassionate embrace. Whether in the name of peace or war, attachment and aversion are toxic and will taint any method of intervention.

If the leader of a nation decides to go to war, people on both sides of the conflict will die. His responsibility for many deaths, or even one or two, will have serious karmic consequences. Today he might be sitting in a big chair, a very powerful man, but in future lifetimes he will suffer intensely. Knowing this, we feel compassion for him. If we truly feel equal compassion for war-makers and war victims, we can begin to embody the qualities of good heart that will inspire positive transformation in the minds of others.

Good heart is the medicine that heals all conflict, the great antidote to selfishness and the problems that stem from it. It naturally gives rise to understanding and compassion; it makes us more open to listening, more able to see why we are having interpersonal problems and how to resolve them. As we give rise to good heart, we watch our own and others' happiness grow.

The great Buddhist scholar and master Shantideva said that awakening good heart is like finding a precious gem in a mound of filth. Once we discover it in the ash heap of our mental poisons, we should never lose or disregard it. Just by hearing about or acknowledging it for an instant, we receive the blessings of enlightened beings. Like the first light of the rising sun, it is the dawn of spiritual practice.

To bring forth good heart, we must use spiritual methods. We are never too old or too young to do so. One of the key points of these teachings is that everyone can apply them.

We begin by cultivating pure motivation. Contemplating the experiences of those caught in cycles of suffering, we give rise to compassion and the aspiration to do whatever we can to help. But we need more than the wish to benefit. We may want to save a drowning person, but if we can't swim or don't have a boat or rope, we won't be of much use. We must learn to swim before we can save others. With the love and compassion now in our hearts, we might be able to help ten, twenty, a thousand, or maybe a hundred thousand people. But even that is not sufficient, for countless beings suffer in every moment. Despite our good intentions, our ability to help others is limited. Any positive impact we have will be temporary, because our spiritual capacity is so meager. We need to dedicate ourselves to expanding that capacity, to fully realizing our inherent positive qualities.

Our true nature is a state of perfection imbued with wisdom, compassion, and the potential to create limitless benefit. For most of us, this nature is obscured, like a crystal encased in stone. We aren't omniscient and haven't completely developed our compassion and ability to help. However, through spiritual practice we can fully actualize these qualities.

Wisdom includes a range of knowing—from the intellect's ability to learn, change, and mature, to omniscience and the realization of our true nature. We all have access to compassion and loving kindness to different degrees; no one is totally devoid of them. Most people find it easy to love their children, friends, parents, or those close to them. Others have a larger vision that includes the desire to end the suffering of all beings. Increasing our love and compassion can be a goal for all of us, regardless of our spiritual tradition. Compassion and wisdom give rise to the power of ceaseless benefit. By applying spiritual methods to change our own mind, we develop an ever-greater ability to serve others.

If the crystal represents our perfect nature, and the stone the negative habits that obscure it, then as we chip away at the stone using spiritual tools, the lucent and beneficial aspects of the crystal will become increasingly apparent. Moments of intuition or psychic abilities are examples of this. Through spiritual practice, great masters have removed all obscurations, fully manifesting their wisdom, compassion, and ability to benefit beings temporarily and ultimately. Enlightenment is the crystal revealed, its capacity to refract light and cast rainbows complete and effortless.

The Buddha left our human realm a long time ago, but we still receive blessings when we think of or pray to him. Jesus lived centuries ago, but his example of love and compassion helps people directly, here and now. Mahatma Gandhi's life was taken from him, but his loving kindness and philosophy of nonviolence continue to influence others.

The lives of many contemporary bodhisattvas exemplify the path of selfless service as well. A great lama in my family, Tulku Arik, went into retreat at the young age of eleven or twelve and remained there until he was about twenty-five. He then spent one year at a monastery, and eventually returned to retreat, emerging only occasionally to beg for food.

Due to his extraordinary meditative accomplishment, his qualities became apparent, and people came from long distances to receive his blessings. For one week every three years, he would let people sit with him. They could see him just for a moment, and only if they had agreed to give up all forms of killing, including smoking, hunting, and fishing. Everyone came to regard the region surrounding his retreat site as a peaceful sanctuary for all beings, including animals. As word of his kindness and realization spread, people began making pilgrimages to his hillside and leaving offerings, which he scarcely touched. He would take only a little grain from a huge sack and leave the rest for the community of poor who had congregated in the area, living off the offerings intended for him. He never accepted money; he didn't own a change of clothes.

In 1959, when the Chinese were imprisoning lamas and searching for members of the Tibetan resistance, they found Tulku Arik in retreat. They bound his hands, tied him behind a horse and rider, and led him to jail. He was elderly by then, very thin, and unable to keep up. Whenever he fell, he was dragged. In a village along the way, the people immediately recognized him. Though it was dangerous to show devotion for a lama, the villagers nonetheless ran to him, crying and bitterly criticizing the Chinese. When they tried to attend to his wounds, he said, "Please, don't worry about me. Help the soldier who is holding this rope. He has blistered his hands dragging me."

The jails were staffed by the most frightening of the Chinese and their Tibetan allies. These Tibetan collaborators, angry with their own people, tortured the lamas. On the first day of Tulku Arik's imprisonment, the guards were vicious, but he met their ferocity with such gentleness that, by the next day, they began to treat him and the other prisoners more kindly. Just being near him, his captors were transformed. Among the prisoners were political detainees who had many grievances against the Chinese, as well as hardened criminals whose anger seethed at inmate and guard alike. By his example, Tulku Arik—though old and feeble—saved them from the torture of their own poisonous emotions, and conditions improved on both sides of the bars. Eventually, a prison once known for its brutality became an exception to the rule.

Over time, Tulku Arik was moved from prison to prison, and wherever he went, compassion followed. This was not lost on the Chinese, who ultimately released him, saying, "This kind of lama is okay." Such is the influence of a person with good heart and pure motivation.

This quality of good heart is the essence of the bodhisattva vow in the Buddhist tradition—the commitment to free all beings from suffering, bring about their unending happiness, and undertake spiritual methods that will enable us to do so. The foundation of this vow is bodhicitta, the compassionate wish to attain enlightenment in order to bring all beings to that same state. In essence, bodhicitta means that self-clinging and self-interest give way to unceasing concern for others.

Someone who has given rise to bodhicitta even for an instant is no longer ordinary. Rather, she delights and becomes a child of the buddhas, for there is no greater service we can render or offering we can make to enlightened beings than bodhicitta.

The ideal motivation, then, for receiving these teachings and putting them into practice is to fully reveal our true nature so that we may be of limitless benefit. Such motivation is selfless, pure, and exalted. The more we bring it to everything we do, the greater the scope and power of our actions. Tibetans have a saying: "The dancer must follow the beat of the drum." Upholding pure motivation in our lives lends beauty, power, and inspiration to the dance, and ensures true and lasting benefit.

The Bodhisattva Peace Training offers extensive tools for doing exactly this. It is meant to serve as a mirror with which to examine ourselves—our motivation, impulses, and conduct—not as a window through which we might judge others. We need to assess and transform ourselves so that we come to recognize our true nature and perfect its expression in our thoughts, words, and actions.

This training is not based on blind faith. Nor can it succeed unless we have a deep understanding of its principles—something we can achieve only by thoroughly contemplating the teachings. So do ask questions. That is your job. It is the teacher's job to try to answer them and make the teachings accessible, fully applicable to you and your life.

TYLER: If we have attachment, we won't be effective, if I understand what you're saying. But isn't attachment sometimes useful?

RINPOCHE: Some kinds of attachment—such as attachment to benefiting others—can be useful, of course, but selfish attachment never is. Sooner or later, thoughts such as "I like this," "I need this," or "I want this" will cause problems. The extent to which we value and cling to something determines the degree to which we'll suffer if we lose it. Someone who knows what a large piece of gold is worth will feel terrible if it is stolen. Someone who sees it as just another stone won't mind losing it.

Wars break out when people are attached to their countries or ideologies. Conflict usually arises in families and communities because someone thinks his way is best. Like icebergs colliding, one "me" crashes into the next.

At first, we cannot completely give up all self-centered thoughts, but we can expand the mind, changing our focus to include the happiness of others. We can ask ourselves, "How can I help this or that person find happiness? Perhaps I have something to offer."

We need to realize that everyone suffers; we aren't the only ones. All human beings face sickness, old age, and death. Many are victims of war and famine. Others look endlessly for something to fulfill them, yet don't know how to find it. Blaming, fighting, harming—people act at cross-purposes to their desire for happiness. Feeling compassion for them, without judgment, we strive to find ways to protect them from the consequences of their actions.

The more compassion we feel, the more we reduce our selfish attachment and purify our karma and obscurations. We become less angry, our mind more expansive. Ultimately, we reduce our own suffering by benefiting those around us.

A CHANGE OF HEART

Compassion and attachment to others' happiness purify self-centeredness—the source of all our problems. Using our attachment to helping others in order to transform attachment to ourselves, we will eventually come to have no attachment at all.

HELEN: You said that these teachings are meant to serve as a mirror instead of a window. If I find fault with someone, should I look at myself to see if my understanding is wrong? Should I ignore my perceptions? At the core of it, how and when do I act if someone is really causing problems?

RINPOCHE: Ask yourself why you are focusing on someone else to begin with. If you are just being critical, then the fault lies in your own mind. But if you realize that this person is making things difficult for himself and everyone else, and you are trying to prevent him from doing so, then your intention is compassionate and your motivation pure.

In one of his lifetimes, the Buddha was a bodhisattva who worked as a ferryman. Once, his ship was transporting five hundred merchants, selfless bodhisattvas dedicated to serving others. An infamous robber came on board, threatening to kill the merchants and steal everything they had.

The ferryman thought, "If this robber kills these bodhisattvas, he will suffer for eons in the hell realms. If I kill him first, not only will I save the bodhisattvas, but I will also prevent him from creating terrible karma and reaping the consequences. I will remain in hell for a shorter time than he would for killing five hundred bodhisattvas. For everyone's sake, I will accept this suffering." With that motivation, he killed the thief.

In the ferryman's act of killing, there was not a trace of self-ishness, no thought of being repaid or of making a name for himself. Because there was only selflessness and compassion, he didn't go to hell but instead created great virtue. The difference between virtue and nonvirtue can't always be seen from the outside. It all comes down to intention.

ORLIN: What if, instead of realizing that they had been saved by the ferryman, the five hundred merchants had accused him of committing a terrible act? Then the good deed would have led to punishment.

RINPOCHE: Things happen that way sometimes. But if you truly wish to help someone, it is important to act. If you are always concerned about the consequences, you won't accomplish anything. Regardless of what others think, keep going. As long as your motivation is selfless, you won't create nonvirtue.

DARYL: Today the ferryman would probably go to prison, or might even be executed, because no one would understand his motivation.

RINPOCHE: Even if he were executed, he would have no regret, because he would have spared both the thief and the merchants. If we have no pride or self-clinging, we will never regret benefiting others. The important thing is to act solely out of compassion.

SARAH: In the notion of pure-hearted motivation to help and protect others, is there any place for protecting ourselves? Can we consider our private needs at all?

RINPOCHE: Yes, in the sense that working for the benefit of others protects us personally from the consequences of selfish actions. But in another sense, our finely tuned mechanism of self-protection and self-preservation is based on impure motivation. To "protect" means to hold on to what we've got. Holding on to self is exactly what fuels suffering. It doesn't protect at all. It actually places us in great peril.

Many people in the healing professions have asked me how to protect themselves from their patients' illnesses and negative energy. I know from my own experiences as a physician in the Tibetan tradition that the selflessness required to heal someone can result in a transfer of energy so that the healer temporarily manifests the patient's symptoms. This is not a problem, but rather an indication of the healer's effectiveness. If she understands this, the impulse to protect herself won't arise. But if she becomes concerned about taking on her client's symptoms, then her fear, self-interest, and impulse toward self-preservation will attract negativity.

The motivation of enlightened beings is one of selfless concern for others, whereas that of ordinary beings is basically one of "me" and "mine"—a little bit of helping, but a lot of self-cherishing and self-preservation. That approach merely results in one kind of suffering after another. So selflessness is ultimately our greatest protection.

ORLIN: What about self-protection on a national level? Are we justified in trying to protect our country from aggression? This is a pressing question right now.

RINPOCHE: If you act with attachment to your country and aversion toward another, you will only create more suffering. If instead you act out of equal compassion for a potential aggressor and for those who might die or be harmed by that aggressor, you will benefit everyone equally. Act not because certain people are enemies, but because you wish to avert a tragedy that will be catastrophic for all concerned.

ORLIN: If I were to give up my life for my country or family, would that be the ultimate act of pure motivation?

RINPOCHE: If you gave up your life with the genuinely selfless intention to help others, and without attachment or aversion, in your next lifetime you would be immeasurably more capable of benefiting beings, because such an act results in tremendous purification of karma and creation of virtue. But, generally, only someone who has advanced quite far along the bodhisattva path can give up his life without regret.

If we set out on the spiritual path with great enthusiasm and decide to make big sacrifices or commit ourselves to substantial changes in our life without proper preparation, our practice will be unstable from the very start. We might break our commitment later, doubting the reasons for having made it or, even worse, regretting that we ever did. It is much better to go gradually, step by step, so that our good qualities have a chance to develop. Then we can slowly deepen our commitment.

First we need to reduce our attachment. There is a simple exercise that you might find helpful. Take something you value—

gold, silver, jewelry—and hold it in your right hand; then "give" it to the left, saying, "I'm giving this up." Then offer it back to the right hand. From one hand to the other, repeatedly give it away.

It may sound simplistic, but in this small, humorous way, we can begin to break down the habit of holding on to things. We mentally practice giving them up again and again until our grip loosens. In the Buddhist tradition, there are many other meditative methods for diminishing attachment. Right now, it would be difficult for us to give up even one finger. But eventually, after practicing such methods, we would have no qualms about sacrificing our entire body, just as the Buddha and many bodhisattvas have done.

In one of his previous lifetimes, the Buddha, then named Great Heart, was the middle son of a king. As he walked in the woods one day with his brothers, he came upon a tigress and her cubs. She was wounded and slowly starving to death; her cubs were trying to suckle but found no milk. Greatly moved, the prince wanted to help, but had nothing to feed them except his own body. He thought, "For countless lifetimes I have clung to my body, but that clinging has never given me an extra moment of life. I've lived and died so many times, and my body has been cremated or left to rot in the ground without benefiting anyone. At least this time, let there be benefit from my death. I will offer my body to this tigress and her cubs."

He pretended to be tired and sent his brothers to find fruit in the forest. Then he lay down next to the tigress. She didn't have the strength to eat him, so he cut his flesh with a piece of sharpened bamboo and let the blood from the wound drip into her mouth. When she became stronger, he fed her pieces of his flesh until he was too weak to go on. By then she was strong enough to continue on her own. Through all of this, Great Heart did not feel a moment of regret.

At the same time, the queen dreamt that she saw three suns in the sky, the middle one eclipsed. She woke up knowing that something had happened to her second son.

As Great Heart died, he made the aspiration that by the power of the virtue he had created, in every future life his ability to help others awaken to a state of freedom might grow. The earth trembled, rainbows filled the sky, flowers fell from the heavens, and the joyful music of celestial beings resounded throughout the region. With that one perfect, selfless act, he gained more capacity to benefit than he would otherwise have achieved in eons.

Some of the prince's hair and bones are in Nepal in a stupa, a monument that is a symbolic representation of the deathless nature of mind, greatly benefiting anyone who circumambulates it.

ORLIN: When you think about it, how was Great Heart's deed different from suicide?

RINPOCHE: Suicide is an expression of mind's poisons—aversion to life, desire for death, and ignorance of the consequences of that action. On the other hand, Great Heart selflessly gave his body so that others might live. His deed wasn't tainted in the slightest by selfishness, righteousness, or desire for fame and glory, nor was he attempting to escape his own suffering. His was a perfect act of virtue.

Many great practitioners throughout history have offered their lives for the sake of others. I remember seeing video footage of Vietnamese monks who burned themselves alive to protest the war in Vietnam. Even as they ignited their bodies, they didn't jump up in fear or regret, but sat in perfect meditation posture. The dedication and selfless motivation they demonstrated starkly contrast with the act of suicide.

IMANI: I'm on the board of trustees at our university and am just now realizing that in all my years there, we have never made a single decision based on good heart. Remarkable, really, that this doesn't enter into our decision making in the smallest way!

RINPOCHE: Making good heart the basis of your work and commitment is a very important matter. If the root of a tree is medicinal, all of its leaves, flowers, and fruit will have medicinal qualities. If the motivation of the members of the board of trustees is pure, the university's purpose will be fulfilled. By establishing good heart as the foundation of education, you will support the development of positive qualities in your students and inspire them to undertake beneficial activities.

Your students are like your children. Your care for them will become imprinted on their minds and will pervade their lives. They will come to respect you and the qualities you embody. When they go out into the world, they will take this same habit of warmly caring for others.

The universe is full of things we can learn. But we don't have the time to learn everything, nor do we need to. Instead, we can choose to train in what is essential. No matter what your spiritual tradition, focus your intention on how the university can help nurture, in both students and faculty members, the basic human qualities of wisdom, compassion, and ability to benefit, for the good of the university and society at large.

In the Buddhist tradition, pure motivation is considered so crucial that teachers start every lecture by stressing its importance. By constantly reiterating that the objective of education is to develop positive qualities and the ability to help others as well as ourselves, you will firmly establish this goal in people's minds, and good heart will naturally follow.

If you have a choice between hiring an excellent scholar whose motivation is self-centered and one with good heart, it is preferable to choose the good-hearted person, because her interactions with others will be harmonious. If your staff members' intentions are altruistic, their minds will be flexible. They will be open to the opinions of others and willing to change their own positions if they feel it's best for the students and the school as a whole.

When you hire someone, let her know your school's values. Be very clear about your guidelines and principles, including standards for the practice of good heart—humility, cooperation, and harmony. Explain that anyone who is part of the university is expected to uphold those standards.

SARAH: What if I see impure motivation in a co-worker?

RINPOCHE: It's almost impossible to know what someone's motivation is just by looking at him. We may assume that a meditator sitting in perfect posture is a great practitioner, yet he may be thinking, "If I sit completely still and upright, people will notice me. I'll become respected and renowned for my exemplary meditation." Some other meditator may behave unconventionally, and yet his practice may be completely pure and his mind free of attachment and aversion. Only a buddha or a great master can see what's in someone else's mind. We can know only our own mind.

There once was a yogi who developed clairvoyance while meditating in a cave. One day he saw his sponsor coming, so he tidied up the cave, dusted off the shrine, and made fresh offerings. Then he sat back, pleased with his efforts, until he asked himself, "Why did I do this? It wasn't to make a pure offering to the bodhisattvas or to my lama. I did it because my sponsor is coming." Disgusted by his motivation, he scattered ashes all over the shrine.

~

ESTABLISHING PURE MOTIVATION

At the beginning of each day, each meditation session, and ideally before everything we do, we establish pure motivation. We begin by thinking of the person or people we would most like to benefit, and we consider their lives—the difficulties and challenges they face.

Then we imagine all those who find themselves in similar circumstances. We continue to expand our compassion until it encompasses all beings, each of whom suffers at various times to a greater or lesser degree, and all of whom seek only to find stable contentment and fulfillment. We formulate the aspiration and intention to bring them all to a state of unceasing happiness, establishing this as the purpose of whatever we're doing.

If we have a relationship to prayer, we then pray—to whosoever or whatsoever embodies our highest ideals of limitless wisdom, compassion, and ability to benefit—that by those blessings and through our own efforts, temporary and ultimate benefit may be accomplished for all beings.

MIRROR OF THE MIND

We begin by establishing pure motivation—the intention to practice this meditation in order to bring temporary and ultimate benefit to all beings.

Then we observe our mind while imagining or replaying an emotionally charged interaction. We notice the ways in which we assess, categorize, or judge the other person's speech or conduct. Is desire, aversion, pride, jealousy, or ignorance present in our mind? Do our thoughts, feelings, words, and actions stem from self-centeredness? Do we place our own opinions, needs, and desires first? If so, we reestablish pure motivation. Reviewing recent events and anticipating future ones, we continue to watch our mind as if looking into a mirror.

As we become more familiar with this meditation, we can try it during actual conversations, beginning with situations that don't elicit strong emotions. As our awareness of our mind's landscape develops, we will learn to always check for and reestablish our pure motivation before responding.

Over time, as we become able to do so in more and more interactions, we will gradually awaken to the mirror-like quality of daily life. Our ability to perceive our ongoing experience as mind's reflection will increase and elicit more deeply the aspiration for positive change.

3

Equanimity

TO BE OF GREATER BENEFIT, we must develop equanimity, an equal regard for all beings; compassion, the wish that all suffering come to an end; love, the aspiration that all beings find both temporary and lasting happiness; and the ability to rejoice in others' good fortune. Equanimity, compassion, love, and rejoicing—perfected by all great bodhisattvas—are called the four immeasurable qualities. The more we practice them, the more far-reaching our impact will be in this and future lives.

Though we may wish to love and help all beings equally, we continually sort people into categories—those we like, those we don't, and those who have little effect on us, whom we usually disregard. Right from the start, we must address this tendency to discriminate. To extend love and compassion to everyone—friends and enemies alike without distinction—we must come to the certainty that all beings are equally deserving of our kindness and compassion. Our equanimity has to be genuine, not just a theoretical concept, or we will never change the way we relate to one another.

Space is limitless, immeasurable, and filled with countless beings, each of whom experiences some form of suffering. A key to developing equanimity is to recognize that all beings face the same predicament: They all want to find happiness and avoid suffering. Yet their chances for happiness are undermined by their misguided efforts to achieve it. Driven by self-centered needs, they do everything possible to fulfill them, but in the process fail to find satisfaction and often harm others. Every act of selfishness, harm, or anger diminishes their potential for contentment and poisons their future. Not knowing the causes of happiness, beings hopelessly compound their suffering. Not knowing how to eliminate the causes of suffering, they merely perpetuate it, enduring endless cycles of misery.

Our challenge is to let go of our judgments and biases, including the distinction we make between victim and aggressor. If tragedy befalls a relative, or even a stranger, most of us are moved to compassion. But we tend to rejoice when an enemy suffers. We think he deserves it because he has hurt us or "ours" in some way. This attitude not only fails to aid anyone, but also creates nonvirtue. When we hurt someone with our words or actions, or just wish him harm, we actually harm ourselves.

The karmic repercussion of hitting someone, for example, is much worse than the pain of being hit. The mind is a fertile field in which a single karmic seed can produce many fruits, just as a single apple seed can grow into a tree bearing hundreds of apples, year after year. If an aggressor who has acted out of ignorance and confusion does not purify the karma he has made, his pain in the future will be much greater than that of his victim. It's as if the victim is now experiencing the consequences of having swallowed poison in the past, even as the aggressor himself is drinking a far deadlier dose. We need to find a way to help them both.

A Vietnam veteran and meditator related an incident at one of the first Bodhisattva Peace Trainings. Fortunately, he had not been involved in any of the atrocities of that war, but a member of his unit in the Marines had not been so lucky. He and another man had thrown poisoned cookies to children running after their tank. The men thought they would soon be leaving the area, but instead received orders to stay. They were forced to witness the results of their actions as the children writhed in agony. Their mothers ran from their huts and, holding the children in their arms, carried them to the tank. They couldn't understand what had happened.

He later confessed, "Since then, I haven't been able to sit in a room with a child. I can't look into a woman's eyes. I can't sleep at night. I live with these images day after day." He said that many nights he sat with a gun in his mouth because he couldn't bear the pain. His story is a poignant example of how everybody loses in violent conflict.

I saw this clearly in Tibet during the Communist Chinese invasion. Most of those who came to occupy Tibet didn't want to be there but had no choice, having been sent by their superiors. Many Chinese, as well as Tibetans, lost their lives during that time.

The Chinese soldiers had become very hardened. They swarmed into Tibet like ants. The Tibetan people had no chance; they prayed that the blessings of their meditation practice would support them and wore "protection cords" to prevent bullets from penetrating their bodies. The Chinese believed the Tibetans had thick skin because so many bullets failed to reach their mark.

I couldn't blame the soldiers who came to Tibet. The teachings on equanimity and compassion that I had received, contemplated, and meditated on helped me to feel compassion rather than anger. I thought, "Tibet has been destroyed. Hundreds of thousands of Chinese and Tibetans have died. What has anyone really gained? Everybody has lost. Many people have been killed, many temples destroyed. Only suffering has come of this."

I thought of the leaders who had decided to invade Tibet, those responsible for so much death and destruction. I thought of the karma they had made, and I knew that their suffering would be far greater than anything the Chinese soldiers and Tibetans had experienced. I saw that there was no one to be angry with, that everyone's lives had been or would be damaged.

Another way I learned to develop equanimity was to contemplate the Buddha's teaching that throughout the infinite cycles of rebirth, all beings—limitless in number—have been our mother or father. There are no real strangers anywhere; we have previously been as intimate with every being—not just once, but many times—as we have been with our own mother in this life. No matter what role someone plays now, that being has at one time been our parent.

All of us are like actors in a play who have forgotten who we really are, so we perceive each other as enemies or friends. Once we understand this, whether people are intimates or strangers, pretty or ugly, likable or not becomes irrelevant. Instead of categorizing people, we can learn to overcome the limits of our compassion and treat all beings with the same loving kindness, responding to everyone we encounter with patience and compassion rather than anger or attachment.

To fully appreciate what others have done for us throughout our many lifetimes, we need to contemplate our parents' kindness. Above all, our relationship with them is exalted because they gave us a human body, which is priceless and irreplaceable. When facing death, even the richest person on earth can't buy a new one. The body given us by our parents provided a haven from the torment of the *bardo*—the intermediate state between death and rebirth—where, in a "mental body," we were blown about by the winds of karma. Our mother carried us for nine months, enduring sickness and hardship to offer us life.

Had she simply given birth to us and let us be, we would have died. Humans don't grow like weeds, flourishing without care. We are very fragile, and many conditions are necessary to ensure our survival. Our parents made sure we were fed and protected. Today, if someone saved us from being hit by a car or pulled us out of a burning building, we would be extremely grateful. But we have forgotten that our parents saved us from death every day—from falling down stairs, playing with matches, or drinking toxic substances.

Now we are appreciative if a friend takes us out to dinner or even gives us a cup of tea. But we take for granted that our parents fed us every day. We are grateful when someone carts our luggage, but our parents carried us around and served us for years. How many times did they bathe us, change our clothes, and feed us? How much does it cost today to have someone clean or cook for us? If we calculated the cost of our parents' care—the years of providing meals, clothing, shelter, protection, and training—how much would we owe them? The quality of their love and care was often beyond measure. If we had a fever or didn't come home on time, they wouldn't sleep until we recovered or walked in the door. Even now, our parents worry about us, but we don't appreciate their concern. Instead, we often consider it meddling.

We may think we are very intelligent—more intelligent than our parents. Yet there was a time when they had to teach us everything: how to walk, talk, and even eat. Had they not insisted we go to school, many of us would not have received any education at all.

Finally, this body that is a gift from our parents is a perfect vehicle for spiritual practice. Animals cannot follow a spiritual path. However strong and magnificent, an elephant cannot do spiritual practice. However proud and dominant, a lion cannot meditate. However splendid, a peacock cannot engage in peace training.

Our parents may have been irritable or abusive, but we didn't know or understand what they were going through. We couldn't see the depth of their love or the causes of their conduct. We will never really understand our parents until we ourselves become parents. And by then it may be too late.

Acknowledging the unparalleled kindness of our parents—of every being throughout eons of lifetimes—we aspire to repay that kindness in every way possible. If our mother suddenly developed a mental disorder, no longer recognized us, and became very hostile, we wouldn't abandon her, no matter how outrageous or difficult her behavior. We might think she was deluded, even a little crazy, but our love would sustain the relationship. If our baby were to bite us, we would still love him. We would also love our two children equally, even though one might be compassionate, sweet, and helpful and the other grumpy, ill-behaved, and given to smashing bugs.

If we understand the kindness once shown us by all beings, no matter how their delusion and confusion manifest at present, we will not abandon them. If an aggressive stranger approaches us in the supermarket, instead of trying to avoid him, we will feel compassion. When someone makes us angry, instead of thinking we have the right to be rude, we will remember that she is a former parent with no way of remembering who we are. In defrauding or stealing from us, someone may think he is being clever, but we will know that he doesn't realize he is committing a crime against someone as dear to him as his own parent.

The third and most profound way of developing equanimity is to recognize that the true nature of each and every being is a state of absolute purity. Ideas of self and other, good and bad, what we like and don't like—these are all concepts of the ordinary mind. They arise from the dualistic process of differentiating, judging, labeling, fixating on labels, and investing artificial distinctions with truth.

Our ordinary mind is impermanent. It is not the same as it was when we were six months old. Even now, it continuously changes. If somebody praises us, we feel pleased and confident. If somebody insults us, we become angry. That anger branches out like tributaries of a river, and we relive memories, rehearse our anger, and react by creating more harm. The initial stimulus and its many tentacles of impulse, action, and reaction in the mind are all impermanent.

The true nature of mind is the continuity beneath this never-ending flux, like the white space on a page; the concepts and emotions that arise in the mind are like the words. We experience and identify with our thoughts and feelings, but there is some ground, or openness, from which they arise and to which they return. That openness is the nature of mind.

The nature of mind cannot be found or proven to exist in a literal sense, as if it were a material object. So we cannot say that it exists. Nor can we say that because we cannot find it, it does not exist. Thoughts that it both exists and does not exist, or neither exists nor does not exist, are only concepts; they cannot catch what lies beyond concept.

To better understand this, when a thought arises we can ask ourselves, "Where did that thought come from? Where did it go? What is its nature?" If we examine thoughts, we won't find anything permanent or substantial. In fact, we will find nothing existent at all. This is why we say that the nature of our thoughts—whether positive or negative, happy or sad—is "empty." This does not mean, however, that nothing is there, because thoughts continue to arise. In a relative sense they are true, though the absolute truth is that they are empty. The true nature of thought, of mind, of every being, of all phenomena is empty, yet fully evident.

Emptiness is the absolute truth of all phenomena, the great equalness of all appearances. We cannot call it "oneness" because of the infinite variety of phenomena that occur. Nor can we say that there is only infinite variety, because in their essence— emptiness—all phenomena are the same. This essence defies all concepts of one or many, existence or nonexistence.

The absolute truth is beyond words and ideas. Trying to understand it conceptually is like trying to catch water with a fish net. The net of concept can only capture concept. To perceive phenomena directly, without the overlay of concepts and the dichotomy of subject and object, is to see their true nature.

ANGELA: How do we know that all beings have previously been our parent? The Buddha said so, but how do we really know?

RINPOCHE: If a schoolchild hears a scientist explain the solar system, she is likely to say something like, "I don't understand. How do I really know the earth circles the sun?"

The scientist might find it difficult to convince her with words alone, but if the child goes through a gradual process of learning and contemplation, she will eventually understand. Similarly, if you practice diligently to remove the confusion that obscures the knowing quality of your mind, you will come to understand the interdependence of all beings.

If a spiritual teacher says that something is true, we don't have to believe it in order to benefit from hearing or thinking about it. When we contemplate something we've heard, our mind broadens. When we bring it fully into meditation, our confusion dissipates and the truth becomes obvious. So it is good to discern for ourselves whether something is true and not just accept it on someone else's word.

Our ordinary mind is like a shell of delusion that obscures our essential nature. By removing the shell, we become omniscient, with complete realization of the absolute truth and knowledge of all details of past, present, and future. Those who have accomplished this have taught that if we could see as they do, we would know that every being has been our parent.

ANGELA: This whole idea hinges on a belief in reincarnation. I'm sorry, but I'm skeptical about this.

RINPOCHE: All we know now is this life. One thing that hinders our memory of past lifetimes is our preoccupation with our busy lives. We're so deeply involved in this present existence that we can't remember what has passed before. But the body is like a rented house that we temporarily inhabit. If you could see the truth, you would know that you have had too many lifetimes to count.

This can be difficult to accept, but simply because we can't remember our past lives doesn't mean they didn't happen. Denying the possibility that they occurred is like getting drunk at a wedding, waking up the next day with no recollection of the ceremony, and concluding that it never took place. Just as certainly as today exists, yesterday existed, and tomorrow will exist. This is also true of the succession of our lifetimes.

Look at the way thoughts come and go in our mind. We can't remember what we were thinking a week ago, but that doesn't mean those thoughts didn't arise. We have a thought and then it fades away. Then another thought comes, though we don't know from where. Then it fades away, and so on. How many thoughts, dreams, and days have come and gone? Like thoughts, many different lives arise from the continuum of mind. No one can prove this to you. You need to experience it through your own meditation practice. As you purify your obscurations, it will become easier to remember yesterday, your early years, and eventually your past lives.

Once, a student of the Buddha came upon a man who was eating a fish and, at the same time, beating a dog away as it tried to snatch the fish from him. On his lap he held a baby. Due to his wisdom, the student could see that the infant the man so cherished had been a mortal enemy in his last life. The dog the man was beating had been his mother, and the fish he was eating had been his father.

Great meditators can remember countless former lives and see innumerable future lives as well. Omniscience means having knowledge of everything, every detail, without distortion or confusion. When our obscurations have been totally purified—

even the last thin layers present in the mind of an advanced bodhisattva—we will be omniscient.

HELEN: I appreciate the importance of cultivating equanimity and compassion. But is it absolutely necessary for me to accept the idea of reincarnation if I want to pursue a life of virtue?

RINPOCHE: As long as you have love and compassion on such a vast scale that you leave no one out, it's not necessary for you to believe in reincarnation. If you can make a fire to prepare some tea without using firewood, that's okay. But if you can't, you'll have to gather some wood. If you don't believe in reincarnation, but go through the process of cultivating love and compassion, you will eventually realize the truth of it anyway through your practice.

VINCENT: Why do we speak of all beings as having only been our parent? Weren't they also our brother, sister, lover, friend, and enemy?

RINPOCHE: In the East, the people we respect most are our parents. It's easiest to practice loving kindness with them because it is they who are closest to our heart. Our greatest debt is the one we owe them. We start with that feeling of love and gradually extend it to all beings. But if your parents aren't the kindest people you have known, then start with someone else—someone you love and respect—and expand that feeling to encompass others. Eventually, you will be able to include your parents. The point is to generate equal love and compassion for everyone.

SARAH: What if the relationship we had with our parents was terrible?

RINPOCHE: Even if they were neglectful or abusive, they still gave you a human body, which is the greatest gift we can give someone. Such generosity goes beyond ordinary concepts of kindness. We couldn't even think about our eyes and nose if we had no head. In the same way, the fact that we can even discuss a parent's abusiveness is due to that parent's kindness, for without our parents we wouldn't exist.

BEN: What if they had no intention of giving you a body or didn't want you in the first place?

RINPOCHE: Whether it was their intention or not, you still got your body. Life in the human realm, though you might eat only one small meal a day, is far better than that in other realms. In the hungry ghost realm, beings live for thousands of years without even hearing of food. That kind of deprivation is inconceivable to humans.

When I first came to the United States, I was astonished to hear people say they were angry with their mother. Of course, mothers are ordinary beings with faults and mental poisons, and sometimes they lack parenting skills, but in most cases a mother's love for her child is incomparable. Our mother may have been demanding, critical, violent, cruel, or completely absent; she may have seemed the cause of all our problems. But if we appreciate her gift of life and try to understand instead of criticizing her, we can more easily forgive her faults.

ALEXANDRA: I have noticed that you and other great lamas remain perfectly peaceful even when there are difficult people in the room. How do you develop that kind of equanimity?

RINPOCHE: Such equanimity is possible when we are neither attached to our own interests nor averse to our circumstances, and when we understand that each being we encounter has been our mother. As we develop gratitude for the kindness shown us by all beings, we begin to see everyone from a different perspective, and the walls between us start to dissolve.

BEN: Rinpoche, I really don't get emptiness. If everything is empty, why worry about our own or others' actions, or even about social and environmental injustice? I guess I don't understand what you mean by absolute truth.

RINPOCHE: The teaching on absolute truth can be very difficult for Westerners to understand because it is so unfamiliar. I sympathize because we Tibetans, although extremely familiar with the mind, are quite unfamiliar with technology. I remember hearing for the first time about the automobile, a box mounted on four wheels that could transport people very quickly. I was skeptical until, at the age of twenty-six, I finally saw one. I was amazed. When I described it to someone, he said, "That's nothing!" and told me about a big iron bird with great wings in which many people could fly from place to place.

The Western world has emphasized mastery of material things. To someone from a technologically underdeveloped society, all of this seems miraculous. To people who for centuries have valued mastery of the mind, it doesn't seem impossible to leave footprints in solid rock or to attain enlightenment. Just as I learned for myself about cars and planes, with diligent practice you will come to see the truth beyond concepts, which now might seem hard to believe.

The two truths—relative and absolute—coexist, and neither can be ignored. Fire, for example, is impermanent and ultimately nothing more than illusion. If we reduce it to the level of molecules, atoms, and subatomic particles, we'll find that the absolute truth of fire is emptiness. Yet on the level of relative reality, we cannot deny that if we put our hand in the flames, it will burn. We cannot ignore our everyday reality even though, in an absolute sense, it is like a dream. Through meditation, we come to the direct experience of the inseparability of the two truths.

In the context of relative truth, the law of karma functions infallibly. Our every action has a result, and we must be extremely careful. But while attending to our responsibilities, we must continually remember that ultimately all experience—positive or negative—is empty. Like a dream, it has no substance, no inherent truth.

As long as our experience is that of relative reality, it is important that we create relative benefit. We respond to relative suffering with relative compassion. We use methods to change bad dreams into good ones, unpleasant experiences into pleasant ones. Yet we mustn't forget that we're not yet awake.

SARAH: So does the Bodhisattva Peace Training affect us only on the level of relative truth and have no effect in terms of absolute truth?

RINPOCHE: If you were inside a building and wanted to get outside, you would have to go through a process to get there. Right now it doesn't seem to you that you're enlightened, so you need to go through a process.

In one way, this example doesn't work because once you get outside, you will realize it isn't any different there than inside. Ignorance, attachment, and aversion create an artificial barrier, the fictitious experience of separation from our true nature. As we apply the methods of the Bodhisattva Peace Training, those obscurations dissolve and the absolute truth gradually becomes apparent.

The methods of this training have a twofold purpose: to make us more effective in our efforts to help others and to lead us to enlightenment. The same practice that enhances our ability to benefit will also bring about our awakening.

~

JUST LIKE ME

We start by visualizing one person we are biased against. We remind ourselves, "This person—just like me—wants to be happy and doesn't want to suffer, yet out of ignorance is working at cross-purposes to that very goal. The actions I've judged so harshly actually result from efforts to find fulfillment or an end to suffering." Instead of indulging a patronizing attitude toward that person, we need to ask ourselves how many times we have done the same thing. We may have acted to differing degrees, with differing kinds of beings, in differing arenas, with differing values, but our thoughts, words, and deeds have all stemmed from the same attachment to our own ideas of what is best. So we see that, out of ignorance, we have been caught in the same counterproductive cycle of perpetuating the causes of our own and others' suffering, even in the quest for happiness. How tragic!

Next we expand the visualization to include others who behave similarly to this person. We remind ourselves that they, like us, want to find happiness and avoid suffering. Unaware of the actual causes of the happiness they seek, they are sowing seeds of future misery just as we have done and continue to do, in each moment, day after day, in the misguided belief that pursuing our own needs and desires to the exclusion of those of others will produce stable well-being.

We continue to expand the content and scope of our meditation, in stages, to include more people with whom we disagree, those with whom we agree, and those toward whom our attitude is neutral, until eventually we include all beings.

As we become more confident in our ability to generate equanimity, we will naturally find ourselves relying on this meditation in our daily life when we find pride, bias, or judgment present in our mind. At times, we will need to remind ourselves of the steps needed to generate equanimity; at other times, we will find ourselves spontaneously remembering that, just like us, every being wants happiness and doesn't want to suffer. But by not understanding that the cause of positive outcomes is the wish for happiness for others and the cause of suffering is pervasive self-absorption, we all work at cross-purposes to our own and others' welfare.

Finally, we open to a pervasive awareness of our shared human experience.

CONTEMPLATING GREAT EQUANIMITY

We begin by thinking of someone we like and admire, recognizing that their positive qualities are like the crystalline reflection of the inherently pure nature of all beings. Then, letting go of the effort to grasp this understanding conceptually, we let the mind rest for a moment in the openness within which we can recognize our natural state, the ultimate great equanimity.

At first, it may be difficult to maintain the state of rest that can give rise to this non-conceptual experience of great equanimity. If so, as the mind becomes distracted by the effort to examine, question, or understand, we redirect our attention to contemplate the possibility that the true nature of beings toward whom we are more neutral is also inherently pure, pristine, and obscured only temporarily by superficial stains. Then, again, we let the mind rest.

We then think of someone we dislike and judge harshly. We also consider that—although we can't perceive it—the true nature of that person is pristinely pure. Our criticism is based on our ignorance of our own and that person's true nature. Then we rest the mind.

We repeat this sequence again and again, expanding the scope of our contemplation each time to include more and more beings toward whom we harbor negative, positive, or neutral attitudes, alternating each time with the state of rest. Ideally, we continue this meditation until we begin to glimpse a more relaxed state of inherent equalness, the true nature of mind.

With practice it will become habitual, as we encounter our judgment or pride when interacting with others, to remind ourselves of the ultimate equalness of all beings' true nature until, over time, that becomes our assumption in every interaction.

ALL MOTHERLY BEINGS

In this meditation we imagine that all beings have been our parents many times over. Even if we don't believe in multiple lifetimes and we find this idea difficult to believe or comprehend, we can practice this meditation as if it were so.

We begin by picturing an "enemy"—we can all recall at least one or two people whom we blame for our own or others' unhappiness—and practice thinking of that person as having once been inconceivably kind to us. What if this person, in some long-forgotten time, had given us life, protected and saved our life, and provided everything necessary for our survival, countless times? We consider that this person who has been so kind to us, whose intrinsic nature is completely pure, is planting seeds of suffering instead of happiness through lack of recognition of that pure nature, just as we have done and continue to do, again and again. How can we help? How can we repay their kindness?

We expand this meditation by degrees to encompass an ever-greater number of beings toward whom we harbor negative, positive, and neutral attitudes. We then make the aspiration to repay their kindness, eventually including all beings equally within the scope of this vast intention.

We continue to increase the scope of our meditation until our commitment to benefit all beings equally becomes spontaneous and pervasive.

In daily life, as we encounter situations and people who challenge our ability to sustain good heart, we can ask ourselves, what if this person had shown me unparalleled kindness in a previous, long-forgotten time? How would I respond to her differently? Asking ourselves this question again and again, in our formal meditations as well as throughout our daily lives, we will slowly find ourselves naturally responding with more kindness and compassion to people and circumstances we have found difficult in the past.

4

Transforming an Angry Heart

BEN: Rinpoche, I just can't see letting go of my anger toward people who are responsible for so much suffering, much less view them as my parents. I guess I really believe in the importance of anger in resolving injustice.

RINPOCHE: Do what you can to help, but without anger. The great Indian master Shantideva said that there is no nonvirtue greater than anger and no virtue greater than patience. Anger never brings benefit, only more conflict.

Most of us aren't accustomed to practicing patience when provoked. We're used to getting angry. Then we repeatedly recall the incident that infuriated us and get upset all over again, creating more nonvirtue and reinforcing our habit of responding angrily.

We are like the host who is robbed during a party and goes on to suspect every guest of thievery. The robber makes the nonvirtue of stealing once, but the host mentally repeats his accusations again and again.

If we're angry and spiteful, always criticizing and blaming others, we will produce a whole world of enemies. To an owl flying during the day, every bird is an enemy. The owl is vulnerable because even the smallest bird will attack it. Our tendency to see faults in others is like the owl's daytime flight. Everyone becomes our enemy. The entire world seems hostile, filled with obnoxious people. We won't have friends or lovers. We'll find no kindness or gentleness and feel no hope. The reflection we see in the mirror will be very hard to look at because the face we're wearing is horrible. But if the reflection is repulsive, we can't blame the mirror.

DARYL: If I give up fighting out of anger, others are going to hold me down because they don't have the same intention of giving up anger. It seems to me that if I do what you say, I'll be held down my whole life by the church, the community, and the criminal justice system.

RINPOCHE: You can still do whatever you feel is necessary to change a situation, but do so with clarity, not with an angry mind.

DARYL: So giving up anger won't prevent me from acting?

RINPOCHE: If I were to tell people that in order to overcome their anger, they should be passive and never act, I myself would be making bad karma, holding them back from helping others. Yes, act if you think it's important to do so, but without anger. A bodhisattva, a spiritual warrior, doesn't retreat from what she knows is right. But if you feel you are being wronged or subjugated, don't think only of yourself. Consider those around you and act on their behalf. And don't just align yourself with those caught in the same predicament as you. Think of the ones who are harming you and the negative karma they are making. Act with unerring love and compassion to uplift, and ensure justice for, everyone involved.

When you feel anger rising, instead of riding its wave, wait until it subsides. Retreat into your mind and think about how you might be more persuasive. At times you may need to speak very directly, with strength and clarity. But by speaking softly rather than harshly, you will lend more reason to a situation.

If anger drives you, you won't be able to sustain your efforts. But if you have compassion for both victim and aggressor, you won't give up. You'll remain consistent, capable, and stable. Instead of losing enthusiasm, you will find your energy increasing. A bodhisattva's approach to helping others is to fulfill their needs, whatever they might be, without regard for her own welfare and never with anger. Acting out of love and compassion is the way of a spiritual warrior. It is the basis of awakening to enlightenment.

A bodhisattva would, without hesitation, give up her life for another. Anger could never produce such a heroic mind. Only deep-seated love and compassion can lead to the heroic mind of a bodhisattva. In essence, the purpose of this training is to help us develop these very qualities.

HELEN: I can feel compassion for individuals, but the system that causes so much suffering makes me furious.

RINPOCHE: What provokes us is not as important as how we respond to it. If we respond with anger, feeling that we are right and our adversary is wrong, we create more harm. Compassion is the only good thing that can come out of any situation.

ANGELA: What about self-defense? If I walk down a dark street and someone grabs me, how should I respond?

RINPOCHE: You don't have to give up the idea of protecting yourself. The important thing is how you hold your mind. Do you feel compassion for the person attacking you—do you want to prevent him from creating negative karma—or are you angry?

BEN: I can't imagine having compassion for someone who is harming another. Why isn't it enough just to protect the victim?

RINPOCHE: Protecting the victim is an important first step, but if we don't feel compassion for the aggressor, we won't have any effect on his mind. We might defeat him in the short run, but if his mind doesn't change, our victory will be short-lived. If we can be compassionate toward the aggressor, he will be more responsive to us.

We must at least eliminate our anger. It would be even better to feel impartial compassion for both victim and aggressor. Remember, we are trying to do what we can to benefit all beings in the long run as well as in the immediate moment. This is a crucial point.

HELEN: As an advocate for battered women, I become very angry when I see what they go through. I feel that my anger inspires me to work harder to protect them.

RINPOCHE: It may seem that we derive more energy from anger than from patience—in fact, we can become addicted to that energy—but it doesn't last. Following the momentum of anger is like having a drink to calm down; we don't really get to the source of our anxiety, so we have another drink and eventually become addicted.

To deal with confrontation skillfully and without anger, we must be able to draw on deep reserves of compassion. We are better able to protect others if we are patient and loving. Inner peace expresses itself outwardly, affecting everyone around us.

If we become lost in rage, we can't help. The energy of anger pervades everything, like a foul smell. Its impact goes beyond the victim, witness, and aggressor. It makes us rigid, too attached to our point of view. We lose our qualities as peacemakers. Our inner peace gives way to the tension of anger. Those we work with will sense this, and we'll be less effective.

We need to offer the benefit of a deeper understanding, a model of love and compassion, to everyone involved. Then people will trust us; we will have more influence and a greater ability to protect them.

DARYL: I'm very angry about the tremendous destruction that is inflicted, not just on humans, but on the earth, the oceans, and the rainforests. There seems to be an urgent need to act.

RINPOCHE: Those who damage the environment cause harm in many ways, and the negative karma they create hurts them as well. When we understand that the root cause of their actions is ignorance, we will feel compassion rather than anger. Although we may act forcefully to stop such destructive practices, our motivation and state of mind must be compassionate. If our mother were about to walk into the path of a speeding truck, we would try to stop her. Ensuring someone's well-being must be our motivation for intervention.

DARYL: If we didn't feel aversion to suffering and attachment to solving problems, wouldn't we become apathetic? Why would we ever strive to correct a situation?

RINPOCHE: To take the example of world peace, the peace-maker is often attached to peace, and the war-maker to war. The peacemaker has an aversion to the war-maker, and vice versa. The objects of attachment and aversion are different, but the attachment and aversion are the same. Whether the dog that bites us is white or black makes no difference. The wound hurts either way.

As peacemakers, we have to change our approach. We need to think about more than trying to prevent the war-makers from harming others. We must also consider how to protect them from harming themselves. They think that war will solve every problem; they don't realize that their actions will only bring greater suffering to themselves and others.

HELEN: Rinpoche, you've spoken again and again about the negative consequences of expressing anger, and it's troubling me. One of the biggest difficulties a battered woman faces is that everyone—her family, friends, priest—counsels her against anger. But when I am helping a woman whose husband beats her, I tell her to get angry. That first step of getting angry seems necessary because women aren't taught to stand up for themselves. If I advise a battered woman to be compassionate, she'll just put up with her husband and he'll keep going until he kills her, the children, or maybe all of them. On the other hand, I have definitely noticed that if she stays angry, her anger eventually turns to hatred.

RINPOCHE: When we feel love and compassion, we don't need anger in order to act. If this woman's child or mother were suffering, she wouldn't need anger to respond.

Anger, as a poison of the mind, has less power and stability than love or compassion. It is like a blazing fire that quickly burns itself out. In a moment of rage, she may find courage, but when the anger subsides, so will her courage. She won't be motivated to find a solution until another incident incites her.

With anger, there is always hope—hope that her husband will change, hope that the problem will just go away. When her anger fades, hope will take over, and she'll end up back in unresolved situations that are dangerous for her husband as well as for herself. The cycle of angrily leaving him and then returning will produce a very unstable home environment, and she may find herself even more at risk.

Loving kindness and compassion don't come and go that way. Like a steady source of fuel, they sustain change. They provide a solid foundation for action. If the woman's motivation is one of love and compassion, she won't want her husband to continue making negative karma. She will understand that staying with him won't make either of them happy, but will only cause more suffering. If, with calm, selfless thinking and intention, she makes a decision to leave, she will stick to it.

In counseling women in the past, I have asked them if they think that patience will work. If a woman tells me that her relationship is basically sound, I advise her to be patient, to back off when an argument arises. However, when a woman is certain that she can no longer remain with her partner, that staying with him will produce more harm than benefit, and that neither she nor her partner is happy, then there is no reason for her to stay.

HELEN: A woman often sees some good in her partner and fools herself into thinking he'll be that way all the time. He may be kind twenty percent of the time, but if she's in denial, she convinces herself that he's kind eighty percent of the time. How should we counsel her?

RINPOCHE: If she doesn't have some clarity about her relationship, there is nothing much you can do. But if her thinking is clear, she can look at the situation with compassion and take effective action.

SARAH: During therapy, I would sit across from an empty chair, visualize that someone I was mad at was sitting there, and beat a pillow. The idea was that if I could get my anger out, I would be healed. Do you think that sort of method is ever helpful?

RINPOCHE: A method like that seems to be beneficial—you might experience a kind of release that comes from getting something off your chest. But it won't produce lasting happiness, because it involves separating "me" from "other" and acting on the attachment and aversion that subsequently arise. Even though you are venting your anger at a visualized person, you are still expressing very negative energy and reinforcing the habits of duality and anger.

For countless lifetimes, we have vented our anger. Were this a way of releasing it permanently, we would be enlightened by now. But the opposite is true. Our anger has only become more strongly embedded in our mind, manifesting as negative experiences that further trigger this poisonous emotion.

For example, an angry man may strike his wife, blaming all his troubles on her. Then she leaves, and he finds a girlfriend, whom he also beats, thinking she is to blame. He kicks the dog and hits his next girlfriend. He constantly takes his anger out on others; he blames them and never examines his own mind, never recognizes that there is something wrong with himself. Because he doesn't address the problem at its source, he can't resolve it. Rather, he perpetuates it. We need to come to the realization through repeated contemplation that anger causes harm. Then its foundation in the mind will begin to crumble.

It's true that if we try to suppress our anger, we will only give it more power. But rather than acting it out with body and speech, we can work with it mentally. Or we can simply let it subside.

HELEN: Many of the people I work with were abused as children and remain very vulnerable to anyone who may hurt or take advantage of them. I've always thought that if a person can express and act on her anger, even a little, she can begin to heal the past.

RINPOCHE: From one perspective, she may feel some relief when she realizes that she's angry about previous experiences. But this just involves revisiting the painful past. Rather than encouraging her to bring the past into the present, help her to go forward. Reenactment merely supports the idea that it is helpful to be angry in the present. It is better not to deal with anger at all than to reinforce it.

If we are revolted by a face in the mirror, we can vent our anger at it by smashing the glass. But if we look in another mirror, we will see the same face. Similarly, we need to resolve our anger, or we will see it reflected everywhere we go. Through contemplation, we can examine whether this emotion is ever justified or useful. Thinking about the suffering it brings to individuals and families, as well as to communities and nations, we can conclude that it merely harms ourselves and others, and cut through our habit of giving in to it.

Although it may prove difficult, working with anger is preferable to acting it out. As you walk down a long path, you might risk taking a treacherous shortcut and, in the process, break your leg. It would make more sense to choose the long way around. By the same token, instead of trying to find short-term release by expressing anger, it is better to go the long way around and work with it. Gradually, you will learn how to let it subside. Otherwise, the pillow you beat might become someone's face.

HELEN: But if someone has repressed her anger for a long time, she may not respond appropriately to a threat. Isn't this a case where anger is useful?

RINPOCHE: Anger is never useful. It's a product of our deluded mind, like a rope that we mistake for a snake. Anger always seems to arise in response to something external. If we look more closely at its nature, we will find that it is empty, illusory; it has no more reality than the snake.

The experience of self and environment in this dream of life is like the snake. Understanding that the dream is not true is like realizing that the snake is a rope. Believing the dream to be true, and responding angrily to the circumstances within it, only makes the dream worse.

In meditation, we learn to resolve anger by recognizing its true nature. Our awareness can radiate through anger—like sunlight through water—without attachment or aversion. Nothing is suppressed, nor is anything engaged.

BEN: Injustice may be dreamlike, but it's very real to the victim and to me as the activist trying to confront it. And my anger at the oppressors is very real, too.

RINPOCHE: Most of us believe we have the right to get angry. We feel free to express our anger, most often with those closest to us. But there is no such thing as the right to be angry.

Our habitual reaction to conflict is to blame someone else. Nothing is right because the government is wrong, our spouse is wrong, our boss is wrong. In fact, the only thing wrong with life is everyone else, and we're going to tell everyone how to make it right. But if our vision is blurry, the only thing to do is admit that what's wrong is our own perception; we need to improve our eyesight. If we had no trouble with our perception, we would see the world as a reflection of the crystalline purity of mind. But because of mind's obscurations, everything seems flawed and we take refuge in blame.

Tell yourself that you need to be more loving, to see more purely. Take a look at your own faults. When others do something that seems outrageous, focus on their good qualities rather than on their mistakes.

VINCENT: I know you're right—everything you say about anger. But sometimes when my wife and I fight, especially when she insults me, I completely lose it.

RINPOCHE: The habit of lashing out lies deep within us all. Our fuse tends to be very short, and it is almost impossible to stop ourselves once we start to explode. If we try to squelch the explosion, it will only implode. We have to train ourselves to prevent the explosion from taking place at all.

One approach is to realize that allowing ourselves to be insulted by someone's words is like being fooled by an echo. If someone tells us that the piece of gold we own is nothing but an ugly rock, that doesn't make the gold any less valuable. If a hundred people tell us that the rock on our table is a beautiful piece of gold, that doesn't make it any more valuable. People may insult us, but that doesn't mean their words are any truer than words of praise. Whether we're praised or blamed makes no difference; it doesn't change us one way or the other. Instead, we should tell ourselves that words are no more than the sound of wind over vocal cords.

We can also remind ourselves that an irate person's words and actions are impermanent. Someone who is our friend today may have been our enemy in another lifetime. Our current enemy was formerly a friend or a kind parent. In any case, his words are different now than they were yesterday and will be tomorrow.

Another approach is to contemplate the fact that there is no benefit in giving power to someone's sharp words. If we do, negative thoughts arise in our mind, and we cling to them instead of letting them subside. We then give them voice, only making matters worse. We may think that by responding in kind, we will discourage someone from harming us again. But responding to anger with anger only leads to escalation. If a fire is raging on the kitchen floor, we obviously can't put it out by piling on firewood. Once we realize that anger creates negative karma, which causes suffering, we will no longer want to add wood to the fire.

When we argue, each of us thinking we are right, two mental poisons are involved: attachment to our own position and aversion to the other's. Both arise from ignorance of the fact that arguing doesn't do any good. With these poisons in control, tempers flare and everything gets worse. Angrily overreacting to irritating situations is tantamount to amputating an arm to remedy a paper cut. We can create terrible karma if we don't have the patience to deal with our anger differently.

Ask yourself, "Why would I do to my wife what she is doing to me? She is going to reap the fruit of her negative actions, and I will too if I react in kind. It wouldn't be logical and wouldn't help either of us." Whatever you are experiencing is the result of your karma. Through your suffering, you are purifying that karma. Be thankful that it is ripening now while you have the spiritual tools to transform it. Rather than making more negative karma, rejoice that this karmic debt is being repaid.

Remind yourself that it's not so surprising that your wife insulted you; she is an ordinary being, not a buddha. You, too, have been known to get angry and say rude things. There is probably a reason for her behavior. She may be jealous and trying to relieve her suffering in this way. Don't lend her words importance by taking them personally. Instead of judging or correcting her, or being careless about her feelings, practice acceptance and compassion.

We always need to keep the goal in mind—ensuring happiness for ourselves and others. With the understanding that anger is counterproductive to that goal, we can change our approach and stop making a big deal out of interpersonal conflict. Rather than fighting with your wife, which leads to escalation and alienation, let her prevail.

VINCENT: That's really hard to imagine, especially if I have strong feelings about what she is saying.

RINPOCHE: Whenever someone confronts us, insults us, or threatens our self-interest, we have an opportunity to respond in a new way. The key lies in the mind, in our determination not to do or say anything that will escalate conflict. Our body and speech are like a great ship, the mind like the captain. If we want to change something, we have to change the mind. Otherwise, the ship will not change course.

Just as contaminated groundwater ruins all the plants growing in the soil, retaliation merely contaminates our own mind. Our anger also poisons the minds of those around us, and they in turn feel justified in responding with anger of their own. We are creating terrible consequences for ourselves as well as for those who have been our mothers.

Anger is like a transparency on an overhead projector. Overlaid on the mind and magnified, it will eventually project the reality of hell. Many people think that the teachings about hell are just a scare tactic used by religious authorities to control people. They think that hell doesn't really exist. In one way, they are right. If you dug deep into the earth, you would never find a place called hell. Yet the reality we call hell arises infallibly as a projection of the mind, a terrifying nightmare, the reflection of our anger and hatred that multiplies like an image in a house of mirrors.

I don't like to talk about hell, because it upsets people. They prefer to focus on the immediate consequences of anger in this lifetime rather than think about its ramifications in future lives. But I am telling you from my heart that all of our actions have consequences. Blinding ourselves to those consequences won't make them disappear, nor will it help us to avert them. Ingesting rat poison will harm us whether we realize it is rat poison or not. Nobody would intentionally create the causes of a hellish rebirth, but we can do so out of ignorance unless we become aware of the effects of our anger.

As humans, we have the ability to work with our impulses. If we know that when we throw a ball forcefully against a wall, it will rebound and hit us, we won't throw it so hard. Similarly if we know that the seeds of hatred and cruelty produce hell, we won't let those seeds grow in the fertile ground of the mind. Beings can suffer in hell for the equivalent of hundreds of thousands of human years. It takes very little time to create such karma, but an awful lot of time to purify it. Contemplating the suffering of hell-realm beings puts into perspective the actions of those, including ourselves, who are ensuring that future right now. Why would we do that to ourselves? Why would we make it worse for others by provoking their anger? Out of compassion for ourselves and our former mothers, we can make different choices.

VINCENT: I'm beginning to suspect that part of me wants to hold on to my anger and negative feelings toward my wife.

RINPOCHE: Attachment to your anger is like an addiction to drugs; it will eventually destroy you. Anger is habitual, but through contemplation and relaxation, it will diminish. Try to imagine a previous lifetime when your wife had a different face and behaved in a different way. She was once kind, loving, and helpful. By alternately thinking about this and the teachings on anger, and then allowing the mind to relax, you will learn to give her the benefit of the doubt.

ANGELA: Last night after the training, I was eating at the mall with some friends, and some cops sat down near us. I instantly hated them because of the way some cops had once treated my brother. Then I realized that I was putting them in a different category from us: we were good, they were bad. I saw that by separating them from myself, I had created my own anger, which was exactly what the cops had done to my brother. That was a big step for me.

But still, my anger has its own momentum. When my rage gets cooking, my heart's beating fast, and my teeth are clenched, it's really hard to remember compassion or the fact that everyone has been my mother.

RINPOCHE: True, it's very difficult to deal with anger once it's up and running, like trying to stop a boulder that's rolling downhill or trying to change the direction of a ball you've already thrown.

What we need is prevention: to look carefully at how and when our anger arises and learn to develop a longer fuse. We know that this is possible, because when we think about an angry episode a week later, our perspective has already changed and we can see how we could have reacted more appropriately.

Prevention requires being very methodical at first. Sit in a room and lock the door so that no one can interrupt you, and imagine different scenarios in which you lose your temper. Review them in light of these teachings about anger. Then, when you find yourself in actual situations that make you angry, your anger won't last as long. As you become aware of how you respond to negative situations, you will learn to pull back from confrontation. Instead of exploding, saying and doing things that you will regret for years, you will be able to pause before you react. You will say, "Aha! Here it is. This is my anger; this is what I've been working with all this time in the privacy of my bedroom." In that short interval, you can choose to respond differently.

You have to be persistent. If you practice this for only an hour or two, you can't expect to never get angry again. Anger doesn't go away just because we want it to. We've had this habit for a long, long time. It's like a sheet of paper that's rolled up and bound with a rubber band. If we unroll it after a few years, it will stay flat for just an instant before it rolls up again. To make it flat, we have to hold it open or even roll it backward.

When you do get angry, don't be upset with yourself. Use the anger as a springboard for contemplating equanimity and giving rise to loving kindness and compassion. Each time you do this, your fuse will lengthen. Your patience will increase. At first, you might become totally lost in rage; it will come like a flash of lightning. But over time, by reminding yourself of the consequences, you can learn not to indulge every angry impulse. With practice, you will establish new habits that will help you when your buttons are pushed.

The degree to which you can reduce your anger and give rise to compassion is the degree to which you will be able to benefit any situation. That doesn't mean you have to let someone spit on your new shoes. It means that you respond as skillfully as you can, with pure motivation and a peaceful heart.

BEN: Saying that you don't have to let someone spit on your shoes seems a little different from what you said earlier about rejoicing in a karmic debt being repaid.

RINPOCHE: When deciding how to respond to a situation that would have made you angry in the past, you can go several ways. Accepting a loss and rejoicing in the purification of karma is good practice, although self-interest is involved in that you are thinking about the benefits of purifying your own karma.

Alternatively, you can try to prevent someone from spitting on your shoes, not just because you don't want to clean them, but also out of compassion, to protect him from the consequences of his action. In some situations, you can do this peacefully. Sometimes, however, with love and compassion as your motivation, you may have to use wrath to snap him out of his negative state of mind or to prevent him from acting harmfully.

HELEN: In our culture, many people associate the word "wrath" with the notion of a wrathful God who metes out punishment without forgiveness or compassion. Do you mean that wrath is directed at wrongful activity and anger is directed at the person doing the wrongful activity? Is that the difference?

RINPOCHE: Anger is a poison of the mind, arising from hurtful, selfish impulses. Wrath is an expression of compassion, of selflessness. In some circumstances, genuine compassion may require taking very strong action. If a child insists on playing in a busy street, you might gently tell him not to play there. But if he doesn't get the idea, you may need a more wrathful approach.

The purpose of wrath is not to punish or harm, but to be of greatest benefit. Wrath can be appropriate when other methods won't work and strong intervention is necessary to prevent someone from creating negative karma. Ask yourself, "Would it be wise or compassionate for me to be wrathful in this situation?" However, you have to be completely honest about your motivation. You can't act out of anger and later convince yourself that you were being compassionate. Wrath doesn't have the slightest taint of anger or self-centeredness, but has a mirrorlike quality that enables you to see what must be done and thus act skillfully. It is merely a display, a method of effecting change motivated by love and compassion. If you become angry, you are only fooling yourself about your compassion.

ORLIN: Does this mean that wrath is not an emotion, that we aren't emotionally involved?

RINPOCHE: When we use the method of wrath, we never lose our foundation of loving kindness. Our mind maintains a quality of stability, just as a dancer keeps a steady rhythm despite a varied display of expression and movement.

ALEXANDRA: Can someone's anger toward me help me realize something? Or can my own anger toward someone else make that person realize something?

RINPOCHE: If your anger makes you realize you need to develop patience, that is useful. And if, as anger arises, you recognize its true nature as mirrorlike wisdom, that is also beneficial.

From the point of view of spiritual practice, someone inciting our anger benefits us because, to attain enlightenment, we must develop patience. We can't do that without some kind of provocation—something or someone who forces us to be patient. If, through love and compassion, you can transform your anger, you will inspire and benefit those around you.

ALEXANDRA: What exactly is mirrorlike wisdom?

RINPOCHE: When you experience anger, there is duality—you, the subject who gets angry, versus the object of your anger. In that moment, ask yourself, "Where is my anger? What is its shape? What is its color?" You will find that anger has no substance. This doesn't mean that nothing is there: your face is red, your breath is short. The true nature of anger can't be grasped; anger is empty, yet it manifests.

Mind has a mirrorlike quality. Many reflections can arise in a mirror, yet they have no substance. There is nothing to grasp, nothing to push away. There is ultimately nothing to accept or reject. When we recognize its empty essence, anger is liberated into the mirrorlike clarity of mind.

Similarly, through meditation, we can start to glimpse the true nature of the other poisons. The true nature of ignorance is the wisdom of the basic space of phenomena, that of attachment is discriminating wisdom, that of pride is the wisdom of equanimity, and that of jealousy is all-accomplishing wisdom. Abiding in the recognition of these five aspects of wisdom, we swiftly achieve enlightenment.

BEN: What is the original purpose of anger?

RINPOCHE: The purpose of anger is to go to the hell realms.

DARYL: But anger seems to be a part of our nature. What happens to our natural tendency toward aggression as we progress on the path?

RINPOCHE: Our natural qualities are wisdom, compassion, and the ability to benefit others. What we experience instead is a complex overlay of habits, anger among them. Anger has been with us for so long that is seems natural to us. But it isn't part of our true nature; it's part of our confusion.

∽

THE CONSEQUENCES OF ANGER

In this meditation, we visualize situations in which someone has made us angry, situations that push our buttons: perhaps we were deliberately misled, falsely accused, or violently attacked. In each case, we think about the short- and long-term consequences of giving in to anger—for example, the speed with which anger can destroy positive circumstances. How might the outcome be different if we practiced patience instead of acting on our anger?

Reflecting on these teachings, we ask ourselves: Is it our experience that anger, be it our own or that of others, calms disharmony and hostility, or does it further inflame it? Does an angry response connect or isolate us? Does lingering anger invite resolution to conflict or does it preclude the possibility of stable contentment and happiness for ourselves and those around us?

What happens to our anger when we try to imagine that all beings have been our own kind parent? Beings get angry, not understanding that their anger ensures their own future suffering and perpetuates the causes of that suffering, even as they yearn for contentment. How tragic!

The more time we spend working on these meditations quietly at home, we will find that our ability to interact without anger in similar situations increases, as does our ability to respond compassionately.

RESOLVING ANGER

As we examine our anger, both in the midst of daily life challenges and when reviewing our day once alone, we can remind ourselves that others' words are nothing more than wind on vocal chords, and then rest the mind. We can recall that the situation confronting us is impermanent, wasn't always here, and won't always be here in the future, and again rest the mind.

When the mind becomes discursive once again, we need to remind ourselves that the purpose of all we're doing is to bring about the short- and long-term welfare of all beings, not just ourselves. Why would we expect others to be flawless when we ourselves have so many negative habits? Again, we let the mind rest.

Instead of energizing our anger, we let it subside and consider how we might respond instead with compassion, remembering that compassion cuts the root of negative thoughts and creates good heart. If it seems impossible to generate compassion, for example toward an adult harming a child, we can try practicing one or more of the equanimity meditations. Remembering times we may have harmed a human being or animal less powerful than ourselves can help to dissolve our righteousness and make compassion more accessible. Having given rise to compassion, again we rest the mind.

If we diligently pursue these different lines of reasoning, over time our habit to anger will diminish and no longer overpower our love and compassion. As our self-centeredness decreases, we will find it easier to let go of anger altogether.

THE ESSENCE OF ANGER

When we are gripped by anger, rather than following its content, we can examine the emotion itself. What is it? Does it have a tangible shape? A form? A color? What is its essence?

Exploring anger in this way, we can discover that it has no substance, even as we're encountering its manifestations. Once our experience becomes less charged and we begin to see through anger's shimmering display, we let the mind rest in the recognition that the objects of our anger have arisen like appearances in a mirror, with no basis for acceptance or rejection.

5

Awakening Compassion

COMPASSION IS NOT A THEORY. It is a feeling, an experience. It is not something we acquire, nor is it created by some biochemical process. Compassion arises in the immediacy of the moment, when we see suffering directly and realize the plight of beings, who almost invariably respond to suffering in ways that will only intensify their tragic condition. A natural quality, an aspect of our own true nature, compassion lies dormant within us and must be awakened. This awakening is painful because it requires us to contemplate deeply the suffering of countless beings. Without understanding their predicament, we cannot feel compassion. But once we truly comprehend it, compassion begins to arise within us and we cannot stop it from flowing.

At present, our compassion is biased and restricted. We feel that some are worthy of it and others aren't. The compassion we have for our family and friends, for example, is based on our attachment to them. But everyone, no matter how misguided, deserves our compassion; we need to expand it until, no longer limited by attachment, it encompasses all beings for all time.

Watch the evening news. Plane crashes, fires, earthquakes, social and economic disasters, war, and terrorist attacks are all horrifying examples of pain, suffering, loss, and death. To give rise to compassion, we must put ourselves in the shoes of those touched by tragedy. If we only watch from a distance, removed and isolated, we will become hardened to the misery around us. When we vividly picture their reality in intimate detail, the compassionate resolve to relieve their suffering naturally awakens.

Imagine a desperate mother dying of starvation in a drought-stricken country, helpless to prevent the slow deaths of her children; parents startled by a call in the dead of night, a stranger's voice informing them that they have lost a son or daughter; a frail and quiet man whose wife, in a convalescent home, cannot remember his name; a child whose playground is a war zone filled with sudden, random, and impersonal violence; a woman who has just lost her best friend to the ravages of cancer. It is not hard to picture these lives that so easily could become our own.

Imagine, as well, the suffering of animals. Every creature values its life just as we value ours, but we are often unwilling to acknowledge this. A fisherman doesn't know or care that the fish wants to live, that the hook cuts and tears. An insect scurries away to avoid being crushed. Domesticated animals can endure lives of grueling labor. Cows separated from their calves call out to them through the night, sensing approaching slaughter. Smaller animals are eaten by larger ones, which are in turn devoured by parasites. All along the food chain, animals are subject to constant predation. Even our pets suffer. They become sick and old, and often die in great pain. They are completely dependent on us; when we leave the house, they have no idea when or if we will return, or whether they will be fed and cared for.

The worst suffering of animals and humans is a thousand times less severe than that of beings in the hell realms. If we become more aware of what it must be like to be a hell-realm being, we will never become disillusioned with our human existence, despite terrible illness, chronic pain, a miserable family life, or abject poverty.

Our own fortunate circumstances become apparent even when we think about suffering in the human realm. We are not dying of malnutrition or watching our children starve to death. Our business may be on the verge of going under, or we may have dry rot in our walls, but at least we are still alive. We can feel the sun shining through the window, see the trees, and look into our children's eyes. We are not on our deathbed.

Even the poorest North Americans are better off than the impoverished in other regions of the world. In parts of Asia, people go for years without a home or enough to eat. On the other hand, in the United States many people experience great stress and emotional imbalance, and the suicide rate is high. We rarely appreciate the quality of our lives, choosing instead to fixate on our problems. If we lose a job or a lover, we obsess about it night and day. A paper cut can completely steal our attention.

Compassion reduces our own suffering by putting our experience into perspective and releasing us from the tight grip of our focus on self. Then we can begin thinking about how to alleviate the suffering of others.

Once there was a yogi, a very good meditator, who went into retreat. In some Buddhist retreats, one meditates and prays day and night for at least three years, sleeping very little. Usually, after some time a sign will appear—a vision or dream—to let the meditator know that he is on the right track. This yogi had been praying to Maitreya Buddha constantly, but after six years still had not had a single dream or received a single sign.

He finally became discouraged and left retreat. As he walked down the road, he came upon a man standing by a huge iron pillar. The man was doing something very peculiar: he was polishing the pillar with a silk scarf. The yogi asked him what he was doing.

"I'm making a needle," the man replied.

The yogi thought, "What diligence this man has! I've become discouraged after six years of meditating, but he is trying to make a needle out of this iron pillar using only a scarf!" He scolded himself all the way back to his cave, where he sat down and meditated for another three years.

But after that time, he still had had no auspicious dreams or visions. Extremely disappointed, he again left retreat and came upon another strange sight. A man standing before a tall cliff was dipping a feather into a bucket of water and brushing it across the surface of the stone. The yogi asked him what he was doing.

"I'm removing this cliff," the man replied. "It casts a shadow on my house, so I can't feel the warmth of the sun."

The yogi thought, "This man has so much diligence in the face of such an impossible task!" Again, all the way back to his cave he scolded himself for being lazy. He sat down and meditated, this time even more diligently.

Another three years passed. By this time, the yogi had spent twelve years in meditation without having received the slightest indication that anything positive had happened. Totally dejected, he left retreat once and for all.

He hadn't gone very far when he came upon a wounded dog, her hindquarters covered with maggots. When the yogi extended his hand to help her, she viciously snapped at him. Deep compassion arose in his heart, and he decided to try to help her.

The dog was filthy. Her wounds were oozing and gangrenous. The yogi thought, "If I clean her wounds, the maggots will die.

I can't kill one being to save the life of another. I have to remove the maggots without killing them." He decided the only thing to do was to lick the maggots, one by one, from the dog and gently set them aside.

He gathered his resolve, closed his eyes, and bent down to lick the dog's wounds, but instead his tongue touched the ground. He opened his eyes, and there stood Maitreya Buddha. "Where have you been?" the yogi exclaimed. "I prayed to you for twelve years! You have no compassion. You never responded."

Maitreya Buddha replied, "I've been with you from the very first day of your retreat, but your obscurations and mental poisons prevented you from seeing me. I was the man at the pillar, but you couldn't perceive me. I was the man at the cliff, but you didn't recognize me. Finally, your compassion for the dog purified the karma that obscured your vision. If you don't believe this, carry me around town on you back and see if anyone can perceive me."

So the yogi lifted Maitreya Buddha onto his back and walked through the village, asking people what they saw. Everyone except one old woman responded the same way: "What are you talking about? There's nothing on your back. Are you crazy?" Because the old woman had fewer karmic obscurations than the others, she saw a wounded dog.

For this yogi, one moment of pure-hearted compassion had far more impact than twelve years of meditation. Many people lose sight of the selfless purpose of spiritual practice. It's not a matter of sitting in self-absorbed prayer and meditation in some remote cave or retreat cabin. The essence and power of spiritual practice lie in compassion and good heart. A prayer offered with the burning aspiration that the suffering of others cease is significantly more effective than a prayer made to overcome one's own suffering. Praying on behalf of someone who is suffering, thinking of her as a representative of all suffering beings, is a potent, compassionate act.

One instance of genuine compassion can purify karma accumulated over eons. The Buddha's path to enlightenment began when he was in a hell realm, an ordinary being yoked with another pulling a cart. Beaten mercilessly by guards because they had become too weak to move the cart, the future Buddha thought he might as well try to pull it alone and let his partner rest. When he told the guards, they replied, "No one can protect another from his karma." With that, they set upon the future Buddha so ferociously that he died and was reborn in another realm. Had it not been for that moment of compassion, he would have remained in hell until his karma had been purified through sheer suffering. Compassion is the universal solvent that dissolves the stain of negative karma from this and lifetimes past.

We don't have to wait for a special time or place to awaken compassion. We can practice it anywhere—as we walk, talk, or drive our car. When we begin to see everyone as former parents who, while seeking happiness, are only planting seeds of suffering, we will increasingly regard all those we encounter with greater compassion, love, and respect.

DARYL: I really can't believe that having compassion for the politicians who decide we should go to war is going to help them, me, our country, or our world.

RINPOCHE: Transforming our world into a peaceful and loving place is the responsibility of each of us. We cannot achieve world peace by relying on those in positions of power to set policy. The root of peace is pure compassion based on great equanimity. To be most effective in the work of peace or any other efforts to benefit, our approach must be founded on unbiased compassion. This itself is a spiritual practice. Any antagonism we feel toward those we disagree with will contaminate our actions and undermine our efforts.

There was once a lama, the head of a monastery, who functioned as administrator of a particular region in Tibet. The monastery's disciplinarian noticed that some local people were behaving very badly. He went to the lama and said, "These people are making a mockery of our authority. Can I reprimand them?"

The lama replied, "That might not be the best thing to do. You won't accomplish anything by being overbearing. Let me try something else."

The lama sent the people some food and other gifts, and invited them for tea. Over time, they became friendly and the lama was able to suggest a change in their approach. They took what he said to heart because they had come to trust him. Treating others in a kind and open way is far more beneficial than taking an adversarial stance, which only produces resistance and animosity.

Developing compassion for someone who is harming others doesn't seem right in an ordinary sense. But in the long run, it will significantly benefit ourselves and others as well.

DARYL: A friend of mine worked with the victims of a disastrous gas leak in India that killed many people. Some of his fellow workers argued that they should deal with the victims' immediate problems rather than worry about penalizing those responsible for the catastrophe. But the kind of negligence that resulted in this accident is all too common among many international corporations. Some people felt that if they didn't make an example of this company, others would continue being careless with people's lives. How do we act with compassion to change such corporations?

RINPOCHE: First of all, check your motivation to make sure you are acting out of compassion, not anger. Next, carefully consider the possible impact of your actions. In any given situation, there is more than one way to respond, so you have to proceed very carefully, very skillfully. You may wish to make an example of this company, but your actions might backfire.

When you act out of anger, you don't have much time to reflect. If you don't think clearly, you may end up causing more problems. When you act out of compassion, your mind is more flexible and spacious, allowing you to carefully consider the potential long- and short-term effects of your actions.

Don't give in to your desire to help only the victims and punish the corporation. At some point, those responsible will experience immeasurable suffering as a result of the karma they have made. If you are trying to create more suffering, your motivation is not pure.

DARYL: What if I don't believe in karma or reincarnation? How can I develop compassion in a situation like this?

Also, I don't want to act out of anger, yet I feel that sometimes anger pushes me into doing something ultimately positive that I wouldn't otherwise do. It makes me get out there and confront injustice. In terms of the gas leak, I cannot let go of the fact that thousands of people were injured or killed. I just can't sit back and let such horrendous suffering continue. It is necessary to take a stand; harm in the world has to stop. I feel that if I have compassion for the aggressor, and try to remember the suffering of both aggressor and victim, I won't be able to act. But I want to act. I want to change things.

RINPOCHE: Who knows what caused the gas leak? Was it the fault of the president or board of directors of the corporation, the contractor, or the manufacturers of the holding tanks or machinery? We don't know. There is something else unfolding here—the ripening of karma.

Clearly, the company was not founded for the purpose of killing people. But many people died, and even more suffered. Consider the owners, managers, and employees who have to live with the knowledge of their responsibility for this death and suffering. Put yourself in their place. If you had unintentionally killed thousands of people, what would you be thinking? Would you be happy?

Suffering is suffering. If you can put yourself in another person's place and feel what he is feeling, you will develop more compassion. If you have compassion, you won't be so angry. When you act out of anger alone, you will be far less effective. Suffering is everywhere, and even if you don't believe in karma, having compassion for all parties will help you act more effectively to prevent future tragedy.

If a cat climbs through a window to drink a cup of milk and the cup breaks, closing the window at that point won't do any good. The cup is already broken. The people in India who died or are suffering from the gas leak are like the broken cup.

Though it's too late to close the window, think with compassion about other companies that may be operating with the same carelessness. They too might kill or injure many people, causing great misery and creating terrible karma. Consider how you might help them avert similar catastrophes. If you really want to take action, reach out to all people equally with loving kindness and compassion, never forgetting the need for long-term benefit.

SARAH: In my experience, compassion and love can take tremendous courage—the courage to make the sorts of decisions that are called for when one is acting with pure motivation. I am thinking about how to help my parents, who are alcoholics, accept responsibility for their actions, while doing what I can to minimize the damage they do to themselves and others, and prevent them from making bad karma. Isn't it best to intervene at some point?

RINPOCHE: In the same way that we patiently persevere in helping a difficult child, we make every effort to help an alcoholic who doesn't want to acknowledge the long-term effects of his drinking and refuses to change. His alcoholism is the result of his karma. Alcoholics often become angry or upset when we try to intervene. Nevertheless, we must do so, but with compassion and kindness, never anger. In the long run, they may benefit from our efforts.

The path of compassion doesn't always mean showing a smiling face or doing whatever someone asks of us. It means continually trying to ensure the welfare of others and never wavering from our fundamental intention to benefit.

TERESA: At the hospital where I work, I'm responsible for my staff as well as my patients. When a nurse is careless with a patient, I try to talk to her about being more compassionate. Though the nurse's feelings might be hurt, my concern in correcting her is for the patient. Am I handling this in the best possible way?

RINPOCHE: The caregiver probably doesn't understand that she is causing harm and making negative karma. You need to protect her as well as the patient. But if you admonish her in a judgmental way, you will only create negativity between you, and within the hospital in general. If your motivation is to help her improve her caregiving as well as to protect her from the effects of causing harm, she will most likely respond positively. Her patients will receive better care, and the hospital will function more smoothly. Everything will improve if your actions are based on equal love and compassion for both nurse and patient.

TYLER: Is "mercy killing" a compassionate act? If a being were suffering and had no hope of relief, wouldn't killing him be the kindest thing to do?

RINPOCHE: If you were a bodhisattva with great realization, it might be all right for you to kill mercifully. There is a story about Machig Labdron, a remarkable practitioner who lived in the eleventh century and was marked at birth with the third eye of wisdom on her forehead. She always taught the importance of total selflessness.

A student of hers came upon a dying horse suffering terribly on the side of a road. The animal couldn't right himself, and crows were picking out his eyes. The student ran to Machig Labdron and asked, "Wouldn't it be better to kill him and end his suffering?"

She answered, "Kill only when you can see a being's karma and can be certain that you are bringing his suffering to an end. This horse is on his way to the hell realms. These few moments of pain are purifying karma that would otherwise lead to far greater misery."

Before you take the life of any being, you'd better be sure that where he is going is better than where he is.

ANGELA: You said that pets suffer because they depend on us. I don't really see it that way.

RINPOCHE: I know this from experience. As a boy, I had a small dog for many years. I carried him in my bag wherever I went. When I was eighteen, the villagers in my area went on a big picnic, bringing their finest horses to race. My family had a wonderful horse that loved to race and always won, but most people thought he was too wild and jumpy to ride. Because I was a pretty good rider, I decided to try. There was a chance he could throw me, so I left my little dog at home with my attendant, promising to return the next day.

The whole time I was gone, the dog panicked, running repeatedly up the hill to my tent and back again. He cried all night long. When I returned, he seemed very happy to see me, but when he sat in my lap, he wouldn't stop crying. It was as if he felt he had really lost me. He ran away crying and that night didn't sleep in my bed. The next morning, I found him at his watering place. He had died of sadness.

HELEN: I'm afraid you are saying that self-interest is bad, that we should concern ourselves only with the welfare of others. I devoted a large part of my life to the happiness of my husband and children, and in the process I actually lost myself. Only when I started to have compassion for myself was I able to feel real compassion for others. Don't we need to take care of ourselves as well and not let people take advantage of us?

RINPOCHE: It isn't wrong for you to love and care about yourself, but from a spiritual point of view, seeking personal fulfillment is not the wisest way to do so. The complete cessation of suffering and the attainment of enlightenment require the purification of all karma, the removal of all mental obscurations, and the actualization of all positive qualities. The only means of accomplishing this is to care for others. So actually, the most effective means of being loving and compassionate to ourselves is to be loving and compassionate to others.

Every step on their way to enlightenment, great beings selflessly serve others, and never to their own detriment. For the rest of us, the need for this or that can be a disease. As our grip on "me" and "mine" gets tighter, the concept of self becomes more entrenched and the experience of the dream of life more solid.

Ultimately, it doesn't matter whether your husband and children appreciate your kindness, because no kind act is ever lost, no matter how seemingly insignificant, whether noticed or not. It is as if the virtue is kept in a savings account that you can draw on in this and future lives.

ALEXANDRA: I've been meditating for a long time, but I still feel bad about myself sometimes. When this happens, I do something nice for myself—like take a bubble bath or watch a movie—and it makes me feel better. Don't you think it's important to have compassion for ourselves, especially when we're feeling down?

RINPOCHE: Changing your outer circumstances won't bring you stable happiness. You might earn more money, but it will never be enough. You may have a lover, but will probably decide you need two, or a different one. You may be beautiful, but will still be driven to have cosmetic surgery to fix some small flaw.

Remember that you're fortunate to be alive now, but death is coming. We wouldn't worry about our nose being too big if our head were about to be cut off. We wouldn't worry about the imperfections of our existence if we realized that death was imminent. Genuine compassion for ourselves is based on the understanding that we need to go beyond suffering. Personal freedom is attainable only through spiritual practice. The best way to have compassion for ourselves is to develop a deep trust in the benefits of practice and to dedicate ourselves to the welfare of others.

TERESA: Which is the better way to practice selflessness—attending only to the benefit of others without regard for ourselves or tending our own garden, sharing seeds with others, and helping them with their gardens?

RINPOCHE: When we begin spiritual practice, it's very difficult to be truly selfless. We start by wanting for others the same happiness we enjoy, instead of thinking only of ourselves. Gradually, the more we consider others' needs, the more we feel that our own are a drain on our efforts to help. The balance then starts to shift. We no longer feel compelled to devote so much time to our own garden, and eventually the need for a personal garden vanishes entirely.

From a worldly perspective, it seems as if we will come up short by being selfless. But from a spiritual perspective, we gain immensely from every selfless act. We're not really neglecting our garden. The virtue returns to benefit us immeasurably.

~

DEVELOPING COMPASSION

We begin by contemplating those suffering in ways that are readily apparent to us. For example, we might think of a close friend or family member who is critically ill, or of the countless others around the world who in this very moment are in the process of dying, in hospitals, in war zones, in outbreaks of disease or famine. We can then imagine our own death—that we're about to lose everything we have accumulated over a lifetime of effort. We can't take any of it with us. Our friends and family surround us, but no matter how much we love, depend on, or are attached to them, in a few moments we will never see them again. Imagining the fear we might then experience, we let the mind rest.

Then we make a resolution, arising from our compassion, to do what we can to reduce the suffering of those caught in such circumstances at this very moment, and then let the mind rest.

We repeat this sequence as many times as possible, imagining what it would be like to be in various situations in which others are suffering, resolving to do what we can to alleviate that suffering, and resting the mind between each contemplation.

Then we expand the scope of our intention to include those toward whom we feel more neutral, and then those for whom it's more difficult to generate compassion, until ultimately our compassion embraces all beings and pervades our daily experience.

If we have a habit of discouragement, depression, or low self-image, we might think this meditation would make us even more despondent. However, it can have the opposite effect and help us to more fully appreciate what we have if, as we do this meditation, we periodically remind ourselves of our relative well-being and resources. We can alternate imagining the suffering of others with bringing our attention back to our present circumstances. We are not dying in this moment, nor losing those we love. We are not starving or about to be killed. Recognizing our comparative good fortune and resources, we resolve to do what we can to help those with less, alternating these contemplations with letting the mind rest. To the extent that we can carry compassion meditation, whichever way we practice it, into all aspects of our lives, we can transform our experience of people and circumstances—even the news we watch—into a profound spiritual path, in and of itself.

6

Loving Kindness and Rejoicing

IDEALLY, WE WOULD USE our short time in the human realm to bring joy and happiness to each other's lives. This is love—the aspiration that others find happiness. The mere assertion that we should love each other has little value; we need to exemplify loving kindness. Recognizing that others need and want happiness just as we do, we concentrate increasingly on their wishes rather than our own. Expressing our love for those we hold close, as well as for those less familiar to us, can make a difference in our family and community and set an example for the next generation.

We can practice selflessness very directly by bringing an altruistic motivation to all our relationships. Entering into a relationship in the hope that the other person will make us happy will produce a very different result than approaching it with the sincere desire to work for the other's well-being. Depending on someone else for contentment makes it hard for a relationship to endure. Instead of expecting others to meet our needs, we should ask ourselves how we can best fulfill theirs. That simple shift in focus amounts to great practice.

If we are genuinely altruistic toward one another and constantly strive to meet each other's needs, the bonds between us cannot be broken. When we work for the happiness of others, they will come to value and respect us. Their appreciation will naturally translate into kindness and helpfulness toward others, as well as toward us. Even if we tried to push people away, they wouldn't leave because they would be so drawn to our loving kindness.

On the other hand, self-interest, self-centered hope, and a lack of regard for their needs will certainly alienate others. Splashing and lunging after a beach ball in the water will only produce ripples that will send it out of reach. Similarly, grasping after what we hope will make us happy will simply drive it away. If we place responsibility for our happiness on others, then almost certainly they will disappoint us. Everything will seem to prove that they aren't succeeding. We'll get caught up in wondering why they aren't bringing us joy, or whether someone else might do a better job. It will be impossible for them to meet our expectations, because what we want them to do is relieve our suffering or fill a vacuum in our life. Loving others means, day by day, considering their welfare before our own and supporting their spiritual growth. This is how we approach relationships as spiritual practice.

Because we are familiar with the needs of those we know well, we can find many opportunities to help and inspire them with our thoughts, words, and actions. Think of how much pleasure we derive from a gentle, meaningful conversation or are warmed by a friend's generosity in giving us a cup of tea. We too can offer sources of simple joy to our friends. Whether or not others reciprocate isn't the point. Usually, we are far too immersed in the idea that if I scratch your back, you have to scratch mine. A relationship will never work if there is a balance sheet nailed to the door. By serving those in our lives with pure motivation, we ultimately serve all beings through the virtue we create and dedicate to their welfare.

If we wish to foster a relationship, it doesn't make sense to do things that will irritate or upset the other person. We can avoid doing something that we know will make a friend miserable. There is no reason to push a tender spot again and again. Instead, we should stick to what makes her happy.

If someone at work or in our family is always angry, we need to be patient. We all have faults. We cannot just throw angry people out of our life. When someone is irritable, we need to let her be, tolerate her shortcomings, and make a point of acknowledging her good qualities. Trying to analyze why she is unkind to us is like digging through the trash and scattering it all over the floor. If she is taking up too much room on the couch, rather than being resentful, we can just relax and rejoice in her moment of rest.

In addition to downplaying others' faults, we must become more attuned to our own. The point isn't to get upset with ourselves, but to admit that there are things we need to improve and then go about correcting them. We should honestly ask ourselves, "Am I kind and considerate? Do I cause harm? Am I antagonistic?"

We are always relating to someone, if only at the grocery store or gas station, and we can make use of each encounter to cultivate acceptance and maturity, recognizing that karma is at play. Understanding that all experiences, positive or negative, are the result of past actions, we can learn to accept or even rejoice in them. Instead of blaming others and reacting adversely during rocky times, we can find contentment in knowing that our negative karma is being purified. If everything is going well, we can enjoy our good fortune, with the appreciation that it enhances our ability to help others. Approaching our lives in this way, we will find fulfillment regardless of other people's conduct, whether things go right or wrong.

We can also train the mind in order to develop the qualities that will enable us to act more selflessly, without hesitation or regret. An effective method for doing so is the meditation of taking and sending (*tonglen*), in which we imagine that we absorb the suffering of others with each inhalation of our breath and send them our happiness with each exhalation. At first, fearing that some harm may come to us, we may be reluctant to visualize drawing suffering into ourselves. But there is nothing to worry about if we practice with good heart. Through the power of our selfless intention, we will begin to see ourselves as a vehicle for others' happiness; any negativity will be resolved and our obscurations will be purified.

With this meditation, we can antidote our anger and aversion, and reduce our harmful thoughts and actions, exchanging them for compassionate and loving ones. This training helps us build a stable foundation for developing generosity. If we practice strongly and diligently, we can eventually give rise to such selflessness that we wouldn't hesitate to offer whatever necessary to truly benefit another being.

Rejoicing means taking pleasure in others' good fortune. This doesn't have to be anything grand. If we see someone resting for a moment in a comfortable spot, drinking cool water or enjoying the sun on her face, we rejoice in her happiness and wish that it might increase. We pray that by the power of our wishes, prayers, and pure heart, her happiness will grow unceasingly. Whether it is someone's moment in the sun, new clothes, nice car, or winning lottery ticket, we are happy for her. We don't give in to envy, thinking, "I wish I had a red car like that one." Nor are we resentful, wondering, "Why does she get to drive around in such style?" When we truly rejoice, we leave no room for jealousy, competitiveness, or self-centeredness. In fact, rejoicing in the happiness of others is the antidote to jealousy.

We rejoice not only when others are happy in the moment, but also when they plant seeds of future happiness; this increases the merit resulting from their virtuous act. We also rejoice when someone on the spiritual path prays, meditates, and creates virtue, and we never do anything to interfere.

Contemplating the impermanence of everything can help us develop this quality of rejoicing. We appreciate each passing day because we are still alive. Life is brief and can end at any moment, so again we rejoice and use the time we have to produce the greatest benefit possible.

Rejoicing is one of the swiftest ways to create virtue. Many sacred texts say that those who rejoice in others' virtue accumulate an equal amount of virtue. Similarly, we have to be careful not to rejoice in, or wish for, someone's misfortune or nonvirtue; otherwise, we will make equal nonvirtue.

Once, a king invited the Buddha and his retinue for a midday meal. On that day, there were many beggars around, one of whom was a very rude boy who showed up knowing that the food would be delicious and plentiful. He went to the tables begging even before the Buddha had been served. The guests shouted at him and, clapping their hands, ordered him to leave. Another boy patiently watched, letting the Buddha and his retinue eat their meal. When they were finished, he begged and was given more than he could eat.

Extremely offended, the first boy vowed angrily, "If I ever become king, I won't let a day pass before I've cut off the head of the Buddha and every one in his retinue." Later, as he slept, he was run over by a chariot, and his head was severed.

The other boy, rejoicing in the king's great virtue, thought, "If I ever become a king, I will invite the Buddha and his retinue to a meal as sumptuous as this one."

In the Buddhist tradition, the merit, or positive energy, of a virtuous act is dedicated on behalf of others, often first to one's sponsor, who made it possible to create the merit, then to one's parents, and finally to all beings.

At the end of the meal, the Buddha asked the king, "Would you like me to dedicate the merit of this offering to the one who has earned the greatest virtue?" The king replied, "Certainly," as he had planned, hosted, and sponsored the entire affair.

The Buddha saw that the king's virtue was slightly tarnished by pride. By rejoicing in the king's offering, the boy had also created virtue, but because his was untainted, it was greater than the king's. To everyone's surprise, the Buddha dedicated the merit first to the boy, second to the king, and then to all other beings.

The boy subsequently traveled to a neighboring country. He arrived late in the morning and stretched out under a tree to sleep. Due to the boy's virtue, though the sun followed its natural course, the tree's shadow never moved, protecting him as he slept.

It turned out that this country had lost its king, and his subjects were seeking a replacement. They decided to choose the most virtuous person in the land. It was obvious to those who had observed the boy sleeping in the tree's shadow that he had great virtue. The boy was made king and, soon after, offered a magnificent meal to the Buddha.

ANGELA: Does loving others in the pure sense you're talking about always bring happiness to us as well?

RINPOCHE: Love is the desire that others find happiness. We may have this kind of love whether or not we are suffering at the same time. Even if we're miserable, we can still wish that others attain happiness. Similarly, we may be fully content and wish that others might share this experience. So we can love whether we are happy or suffering.

HELEN: Sometimes we try to be loving, but our actions can have an unintended, even opposite, effect. We might do things that we think are beneficial, but we end up harming instead. What can we do about that?

RINPOCHE: Your aspiration and thoughtful, committed approach to helping others are in and of themselves virtuous when they come from a heart of compassion. All you can ever do is try, overtly or subtly, and as skillfully as possible, to create the greatest gain and the least harm. Sometimes taking a humble position and working behind the scenes is most effective. Other times you may have to adopt a more controversial stance, or yell and shout. If you act selflessly, whatever you do will produce virtue.

The best way to ensure that your actions will lead to positive results is to cultivate good heart. If you are always kind and helpful, and your actions are based on the aspiration to free all beings from suffering, your efforts will benefit yourself and others.

VINCENT: My wife says that we should always express our emotions. But every time we do, we just end up angry, feeling worse than before. I'm wondering if all this sharing is really helpful.

RINPOCHE: Usually, expressing strong feelings is not the most effective thing to do. Some small benefit may come from it in the short run, but this approach is founded on the mistaken belief that our emotions are caused by someone else's actions. That is a very shortsighted perspective. The real cause of our experience is karma. It is karma that determines the kind of exchange we have with someone.

This doesn't mean that you must accept your suffering passively or fatalistically. You have choices. If you are having difficulties but would like to keep the family together, you can choose to be patient and compassionate instead of hostile and angry. When your wife hurts you, you can choose not to dwell on it, but to simply let it go. Rather than brood over what is painful, you can turn your mind in another direction.

Sometimes it's most beneficial to give in to someone, to give her what she feels she needs. Though it may seem that you are weak or losing out, nothing is lost. If the family relationship improves, there is only gain.

As for expressing or processing feelings in moments of conflict, consider how you feel when someone scowls at you or is critical, cold, and rude. If someone is considerate and respectful, even during disagreements, isn't it easier to respond in kind?

This is an ancient and practical truth: treat others as you wish to be treated.

If you look for faults in others, you will certainly find some. If all you do is berate your loved ones for their shortcomings, they won't want to be around you. When they don't show you their most loving face, remind yourself of all the times you have been less than kind. Just as the storms of our own emotions come and go, the anger or irritation of loved ones will pass with time. If we solidify our concept of them as angry people, then that is what we will see, regardless of their mood.

The key lies in understanding that we can find in ourselves the shortcomings we see in others. We shouldn't cling to the notion that others are primarily at fault, but rather examine our own behavior and how we may be causing conflict. If we continue to talk or act in a critical or confrontational way, we are likely to irritate others and experience even more conflict in the future.

ALEXANDRA: I've had a number of wonderful romantic relationships. Isn't it preferable to keep a relationship harmonious and, when things get messy, when anger starts coming up and so forth, to end it and begin again with someone else?

RINPOCHE: Actually, it's helpful in a worldly as well as a spiritual way to persevere in relationships. This creates a basis for trust and establishes conditions that support your partner in his spiritual practice. If someone relies or pins his hopes on you, don't be indiscriminate with that trust.

If we decide to be intimate with another person, we must accept the responsibilities of that intimacy. Given such closeness, it's easy to upset his mind. If we enter relationships too casually, we will hurt people's feelings, causing emotional disturbances and difficulties. When this happens, we need to reassess our behavior.

Anger doesn't have to be a big issue. When it arises, let it go. If your partner is having a bad day, it is best to ignore his mood. This doesn't mean you don't care, only that the situation may require patience instead of fixing. Give him space. Let time do the healing. If you press to find out what upset him or try to analyze what you did wrong, you'll often make things worse. Because the human psyche is so erratic, it is impossible to resolve every detail. If you don't react to each little thing he does, your flexibility will give him room to change. A quick fix of an issue or personality quirk is usually not very stable anyway. There has to be space to act from the heart. The real issue—and the basis of your bond—is trust.

TYLER: What do we do if selfish desire is our strongest motivation and overpowers selfless love?

RINPOCHE: Contemplate the fact that when we become lost in desire, we perpetuate suffering. The objects of our attachment—people, possessions, or states of being—are illusory, yet we continue to grasp at them like a child chasing a rainbow. Desire is like a lure that, when pursued, eventually produces a negative outcome.

Our suffering is caused not by the objects of our desire, but by our attachment to them. Whether our dream reality is good or bad, it is best to cultivate satisfaction and enjoy what we already have. Though our life may not be the best, it certainly isn't the worst of all possibilities. Nothing is deeply or permanently fulfilling anyway. Although we may feel an insatiable need for more, that new relationship, car, house, or job won't fill up the hollow place in our heart. We have enough food to eat and enough clothes to wear; we have what we need to stay alive. Through contemplation we begin to recognize where attachment will lead us as it courses through our present and future experiences.

Once you have achieved a degree of spiritual maturity, you can work with desire on another level. Look directly into its essence as emptiness and then let the mind relax. Both methods—contemplation and looking into the nature of desire—are useful. Both arrows hit the same target. Use whichever seems appropriate.

ANGELA: In many situations, like walking into a shopping mall, I notice that I feel alienated from others and erect a wall around myself. However, I feel very openhearted with my mother and father, whom I love very much. Can you explain what makes me put up these walls of separation so much of the time?

RINPOCHE: Normally, we focus primarily on ourselves, and this alienates us from others. So, as you have described, when we seek to protect ourselves, we create walls instead of extending all-pervasive loving kindness. Practicing the "Taking-and-Sending" meditation whenever you notice yourself doing this will help dissolve these artificial barriers.

VINCENT: If I try everything you've suggested and my wife and I still can't work things out, would it be better for us to get a divorce?

RINPOCHE: It's usually best to maintain a relationship rather than to let it go. According to a Tibetan saying, "An old demon is better than a new god." No one is flawless. A new relationship may seem wonderful for two or three years, but eventually problems will arise. It will never be perfect. There will always be disagreements.

However, sometimes a marriage simply stops working. In spite of your best efforts to be loving, kind, and compassionate, you and your partner find yourselves miserable. Your anger and fighting place your children under stress, which may cause emotional problems for them later on. In that case, your relationship isn't benefiting anyone. As much as you might like to work things out, there is no point in prolonging the misery. If there is no happiness in your household and you are only creating nonvirtue, divorce may be a better option. However, making such a decision in a moment of anger won't produce a sound and stable resolution. Talk things over when you both are calm and clear.

VINCENT: As I've watched my marriage fall apart, I've vacillated between anger and depression. I haven't been able to find a positive way through it.

RINPOCHE: Like your initial attraction to your wife, these more recent events are the result of your karma. Rather than blame her, remind yourself that everything you experience is due to karma. If there is karma for your relationship to succeed, nothing could prevent it from working. If the karma for being together is finished, nothing could keep it from ending.

If you dwell on your situation, you will become more and more unhappy until, at some point, your wife will seem like a demon rather than the angel you once thought her to be. So don't indulge in negative thoughts; instead, wish her every happiness.

Your depression is the result of your attachment. Remember, all things change. One day you will lose even your body. From that perspective, anything this side of death is okay. As long as you have a body, much is still possible. Redirect your focus from what has been lost to what you still have.

Rather than trying to prevent your karma from unfolding, rely on prayer. Pray for what is best for you, your wife, and all beings, whatever that might be. You may think it's best for your marriage to last, but who knows? That might only produce more suffering.

HELEN: My husband was emotionally abused as a child and is very controlling, something I find hard to deal with.

RINPOCHE: You know he was abused; he has some emotional problems that you've been spared. As a result, it's easier for you to be spacious. Do what you can to maintain your patience, and to help and support him. Be kind and loving, and when he's angry, don't react. Spiritual practice starts with the family.

TERESA: My sister is trying to decide whether to leave her husband, who physically abuses her. The abuse is also emotionally damaging, not only for her, but for their children.

RINPOCHE: Sometimes it is better for children if their parents separate, especially if the children are growing up in an unstable, unloving, or violent household. This situation is not only harmful to them, but provides no positive example for them to follow.

Generally speaking, however, it is preferable for parents to try to work things out.

Ideally, our goal in relationships is to create happiness, not pain and suffering. We are together only briefly before death separates us. Our children are with us for a very short time as well, and then they go their own way. Although our greatest aspiration is to benefit as many beings as possible, we should at least seek to bring happiness to those closest to us, whose lives we affect every day.

We need to do what we can within the relationship. This means developing tolerance for others' faults and, if our behavior, speech, or habits are irritating, trying to change them. But if, despite our sincere efforts, the situation continues to deteriorate—there is still constant blame, nothing we do pleases our spouse, and no one is happy—then it is obvious that everybody is caught in a web of suffering, and we need to act. Even if we haven't saved the relationship, the attempts we've made to change ourselves will support more peaceful interactions in the future.

However, for some people, one violent relationship follows another. Sometimes such violence is the result of karmic links between those who have interacted negatively in previous lifetimes. Such circumstances can manifest explosively. Your sister must think very carefully about what to do. She might consider leaving her husband to protect him from perpetuating nonvirtue. If she truly believes that staying with him will only lead to more suffering and that resolution is impossible, it is clearly best to leave.

BEN: You said that when somebody has good fortune, we should rejoice. But if that good fortune comes at your expense, it's hard to get to that feeling. If my boss is happy because he fired me to save money and I'm hurting as a result, how can I rejoice for him?

RINPOCHE: Loss and gain need to be understood from a karmic perspective. When you lose something in spite of your best efforts to hold on to it, this means that karma is the culprit. Nothing in the world could have prevented that loss. The cause was the ripening of a karmic seed that you yourself planted. As the events played themselves out, the karma was exhausted. In other words, a poisonous seed grew into a poisonous plant, which was the loss you experienced. With that, the plant was uprooted. So more is involved here than just being fired from a job.

If we approach loss or similar difficulties skillfully, we can even gain from them. We can consider, "This is my karma ripening. I've lost this job, but the karma I once created is now finished. I won't have to deal with it again." We can rejoice because we have repaid a karmic debt. On the other hand, if we become indignant, thinking we've been cheated, our anger and resentment will only result in more negative karma.

When we lose something, instead of blaming someone else, we can consider the loss to be a repayment to a kind parent and rejoice because we haven't complicated the situation by making more negative karma. When we really understand that all beings, including our employer, have been our kind and loving parents, rejoicing in another's happiness becomes possible even in the face of loss.

~

EXPANDING OUR LOVING KINDNESS
AND REJOICING

We begin by thinking about our interactions with those close to us as well as those with whom we have only a fleeting acquaintance. How would we interact with them differently if we were certain that we want to use our precious and brief time on earth only to bring joy and happiness to all those we encounter? We alternate this contemplation with letting the mind rest. Then we make a resolution arising from our contemplation. For example, we might commit to become more fully and unequivocally loving toward a particular person or group of people, and again let the mind rest.

We could also take the approach of reviewing a particularly charged and tense encounter from the perspective of evaluating how our own faults escalated the difficulties, bringing our awareness to the other person's positive qualities that we may have overlooked. How might the tension have been diminished if we had validated their qualities instead of reacting to their flaws? How might the exchange have unfolded if we had taken responsibility, inwardly and outwardly, for our own shortcomings? Then we rest the mind. Next we make a commitment arising from this evaluation. For example, we might resolve always to acknowledge others' points of view in every interaction. And then rest the mind.

We might then contemplate how differently that same interaction might have gone if we had approached it from the perspective of wanting the other's happiness and trying to meet their needs rather than our own. We alternate that contemplation with resting the mind. Then we might make a commitment to think only of that person's welfare instead of our own the next time we encounter them. And again rest the mind.

We continue to expand the scope of our loving kindness and the depth of our commitment to love more fully, without hesitation or compromise, until it embraces all beings.

We can also repeat this process as we contemplate the practice and benefits of rejoicing. Imagining a variety of virtuous and fortunate experiences enjoyed by others, we rejoice in their positive circumstances and their actions, which plant the seeds of future good fortune. For example, first at home when alone and then at work once we become more habituated to the practice, we might rejoice in the happiness of someone at our workplace who receives a promotion rather than us, thus antidoting any jealousy, competitiveness, or self-centeredness we might previously have felt.

Or we might rejoice whenever we see an act of kindness, the basis of future happiness. And then rest the mind. Rejoicing in the causes of others' good fortune and in that fortune as it occurs, we resolve, for example, to practice the same kindness and then rest the mind.

We could then try to imagine all the acts of kindness occurring in the world at this very moment, and make the wish and aspiration that such kindness would only increase until all beings know only the unbounded joy resulting from such virtue. And then rest the mind.

TONGLEN: TAKING AND SENDING

We start by envisioning one or two beings for whom we easily feel compassion, whose suffering particularly moves us. We contemplate their misery and put ourselves in their place, imagining what their lives must be like. Once compassion arises, we begin the following meditation with the fervent wish to relieve their and others' suffering and assure the temporary and ultimate happiness of all beings.

Following the natural rhythm of our breath, we visualize that, as we inhale through the nose, we take in all of the causes and conditions of their suffering in the form of murky light, imagining that they become completely free of misery. With each exhalation, we visualize that we are sending and they are receiving all our merit, as well as all conceivable sources and experiences of enduring happiness, as radiant, pure light.

We then gradually expand the visualization to include more and more beings for whom our compassion is accessible, eventually incorporating beings toward whom our feelings are more neutral.

Next, we include first one and then others toward whom we feel anger or aversion. We gradually increase the scope of our visualization to include more and more beings toward whom we have previously felt antipathy, until our loving kindness and compassion embrace all beings throughout time and space.

If we find that our habits of anger and aversion prevent us at times from responding to others with kindness, we can utilize this meditation to transform our negativity, first when alone reviewing difficult circumstances we have encountered, and eventually in our daily lives as we engage with others.

As we become increasingly accustomed to breathing in others' suffering and sending them happiness, we can imagine someone we wish to help but don't have the outer means to do so. From the shift in perspective that comes from this practice, we may even find that we develop insight into ways we might be able to bring benefit that we couldn't perceive previously. Or if we find ourselves in a meeting filled with conflict and anger, we may discover that this practice can help ease some of the negativity present, if only in our own minds.

When we're at home or in situations where we can focus one-pointedly on our meditation, we can rest the mind between each successive visualization. This will allow the possibility for the mind to awaken to the spontaneous experience of limitless, pervasive, and all-encompassing love and compassion.

7

The Heart of Parenting

TERESA: How can I teach loving kindness to my children?

RINPOCHE: The most effective way for parents to teach their children spiritual values is to live them—to demonstrate respect, loving kindness, and compassion. Children don't always know how to behave, so we need to exemplify good heart through our conduct. We accomplish far more by living the teachings than by simply telling our children what or what not to do. If we want to teach the principle of not harming, we must live by not harming. When we are kind and respectful to our own parents and to each other, and when we resolve our problems harmoniously, we set examples that our children can follow in forming their own successful relationships. Children develop a deep trust of the principles we demonstrate to them.

Storytelling is also an effective method. On Sundays when I am home, local children come by. We sit on the floor together and eat popcorn, and I tell one or two stories. Each story conveys a lesson, such as the positive results of practicing good heart or the negative consequences of harmful thoughts and actions. In essence, that is how I approach spiritual teaching with children under the age of eleven or so; I don't formally instruct them.

It's important to be spacious and not attempt to push children into spiritual practice, because if we pressure or try to entice them, they will almost certainly resist. They will, however, recognize sincerity. If we apply the teachings to our own mind, our children will benefit from and see the value of our patience and kindness. Then they will come to spiritual practice because they want to, not because their parents told them to. And if they don't want to, they don't have to.

Children are the future, the ones who will maintain decency in the world. If we treat them as though they were insignificant, become harsh or overly stern, or neglect them because we're meditators who have no time to play with them, they will only resent us and spiritual practice.

TERESA: What happens when my children go to school and encounter different values?

RINPOCHE: One of my students and her son lived with me at my center from the time the child was three years old. When he went to grade school, I told him not to say anything about Buddhist teachings. But he didn't listen. He told his mother, "Rinpoche told me not to talk about the teachings, but I know they help when you die, so I'm going to tell anyone I want."

Sometimes a crisis would occur that he couldn't bear. One day, some children stomped on worms in rain puddles, and he tried in vain to stop them. Another time, some neighborhood children peeked into our shrine room. When they saw a cat sitting on the lama's seat, they came to the conclusion that we worship cats.

Finally, when he was about nine, the boy said, "Rinpoche, we've got a big problem. None of the kids at school understand what Buddhism is. When they look it up in the encyclopedia they find 'idol worship,' so now they call me 'idol worshiper.'"

I asked, "What do you think the problem is?"

He replied, "The problem is that I can't explain Buddhism to them. I know in my heart that it's right, but I can't get past all their wrong ideas to share anything about it."

"What do you think the solution is?" I asked him.

"I think the solution is not to talk to the kids at school about the teachings."

I replied, "That sounds good. In your heart, you know they are something you love and understand. That's what matters."

HELEN: How can we strike a balance between gentleness and discipline with children? We never know if we're making the right decisions.

RINPOCHE: Parenting requires considering how to benefit our children and offer them the best opportunities. We have to assess their short- and long-term needs, and respond to anything they do or say that might be harmful.

We discipline children not for our sake, but for theirs. We must teach them not to argue, fight, or use harsh words. If they don't listen, we have to set some guidelines. If your son wants to play in the street, and you have to keep bringing him back to the sidewalk, it may be necessary to spank him or use another disciplinary method to keep him there. However, your motivation must always be based on good heart.

In an environment devoid of loving kindness, gentleness, or trust, any attempt to discipline children will only make them more anxious, disturbed, and emotional. But assuming that they have developed a strong sense of security in an environment of loving care, if they do something harmful, the use of wrath can sometimes be appropriate. Coming from deep-hearted compassion and the desire to benefit, wrath can help conquer their pride and anger, and avert negative behavior. Discipline motivated by anger won't have the same effect.

This is just my approach, the Tibetan approach. Western children are better educated and enjoy more opportunities for entertainment than Tibetan children. Their parents are frequently very permissive, but I've seen that children in the West often do not have enough respect for their parents. In Tibet, we don't have as many diversions; children don't have an array of toys and gadgets. We're often wrathful with them, but as they grow up, they tend to have more respect and appreciation for their parents. So maybe the Tibetan ideas about raising children have some merit.

HELEN: Some of the kids we work with are very unruly, yet don't respond well to discipline. They have been abused at home. What can we do?

RINPOCHE: That is difficult to say. If parents discipline their children, it's easier for someone outside the family to do it, too. The approach should be consistent; otherwise, children won't trust or respect those who are providing structure in their lives. In Tibet, in monasteries and among lay people, children are strictly disciplined. But they receive the same discipline—and loving kindness—from every adult.

Consistent discipline is difficult to achieve here in the West because we don't agree about how to enforce basic rules of behavior with children. For example, if a child tells her parents how she was disciplined at school and they respond, "What a terrible thing your teacher did," the child will lose her respect for the teacher. But if the parents support the teacher—if they work together—then disciplinary measures can be effective.

In the same way, parents need to support each other. For example, if a father is wrathful with a child, she may run crying to her mother. If the mother responds with, "I'm so sorry. Why did Daddy do that to you?" then the father's discipline loses its power. If the mother ignores or questions what the father has said, the child will, too. If, on the other hand, the mother supports the father by saying, "Be careful, don't do that again. Your father is helping you," the child will respect him. A unified approach to instilling positive behavior and values will be most beneficial.

ANGELA: Most of this sounds so simple and easy to understand. But the important things you're saying go very deep, and I feel that a lot of teenagers won't understand them. How do you teach children at the right age, before it's too late and they've become stuck in negative patterns?

RINPOCHE: Children comprehend so much more than we think they do. They will benefit every time we help them understand the power of loving kindness.

I may seem very peaceful to you now, but as a child I definitely was not! When I was about nine, my stepfather came to live with us. He was a very nice man, but I didn't feel good about having him around because, until he arrived, it had been my house, my domain. I wasn't very happy that a bigger man had taken over.

My father, whom I never met, was a great lama, as was my mother. Many guests came to see her and brought offerings, usually sweets. So my mother always had a big bag of candies—a very rare thing in Tibet. All I had to do was ask, and I could have as many as I wanted. I could pass them out to my friends. The whole bag was mine.

When my stepfather moved in, he used the candies for offerings. The bag was tied shut, and they were no longer mine alone. I was furious!

I devised a plan to kill him. I made a bow and arrow that suited me perfectly. Through a window, I could just see the top of his head as he sat in meditation. I shot an arrow directly at him and ran away. I was sure I had killed him, and was happy to be rid of him, but when I turned around, there he was, standing outside, holding his head and laughing. The arrow had only grazed his head.

You can see that I didn't exactly start out in a peaceful state. For all children, a great deal of life experience and exposure to positive role models can help resolve such tendencies to misbehave.

ANGELA: Is it enough to reflect loving kindness back to children who have been abused? It's hard to imagine this tactic succeeding with some of the kids I know.

RINPOCHE: When a tragedy or crisis occurs in a child's life, he suffers from more than emotional scarring; trauma also affects the physical body. Our insubstantial minds and substantial bodies are joined by a subtle energy called the life-sustaining wind. When someone experiences great fear, anxiety, or sadness, this energy becomes unbalanced, almost as if something had popped out of place. It is often precipitated by terror—life-and-death situations such as accidents or brutal beatings—but the imbalance can result from something seemingly harmless as well, such as when a child scares a sibling while at play. Although the mind-body connection is immediately restored, the subtle energy stays slightly out of kilter. This is similar to quickly opening and closing the lid on a vacuum-packed jar. The contents of the jar may appear as before, but the seal has been broken. Over time, the impact on the contents becomes apparent.

As we get older, and issue piles upon issue, our subtle energy becomes increasingly disturbed. Many people I've met in the United States suffer from this imbalance. To help people with emotional problems, we must address the physical imbalance as well as the emotional scars. Methods for treating the physical component include eating small portions of cooked, rather than raw, food (ideally animal products) prepared with oil, and doing so regularly and frequently. It also helps to take baths rather than showers, put oil in the bathwater and on the skin, establish patterns of regular and adequate sleep, and reduce stress and pressure. Then spiritual teachings and contemplation can more easily address the emotional component.

HELEN: Rinpoche, do you have any specific advice about working with teenagers?

RINPOCHE: We need to be especially patient with teenagers because trying to discipline them won't really work. We can help them most by supporting them and sharing our ideas about what might be helpful, rather than trying to control their personal lives. When they're not caught in the middle of a difficult problem or upheaval, we can assist them in exploring the possible effects of their actions, as well as discuss the choices they are contemplating for their future. My experience is that if we are too strict with teenagers, they will simply resist. If we're open and supportive, they will feel freer to talk about their problems.

HELEN: I have two daughters. One is thirteen, the other ten. My older daughter has always been jealous of her sister and is very mean to her. How should I handle this?

RINPOCHE: It's too late to try to discipline the older daughter. The time to start disciplining children is when they are young, from about three to eight years old. When they are older, it's more difficult to change their habits.

Once the time for disciplining children has passed, it is best to be kind and patient with them so they don't perceive you as their enemy. Being overly critical won't help. Rather, praise can soften children at this age. You might say to your daughter, "You're doing really well. Maybe you would find that if you did such and such, things would go even better." You can also try to talk to her openly.

When I was young, I also was cruel to my sister. I even struck her sometimes. Then, when I was eleven and she was two, our mother died. My tutor said to me, "Why do you treat your sister like this? Now that your mother is gone, you're the only family

THE HEART OF PARENTING

she has. She needs you and loves you so much." I thought about what he had said and cried. My sister was young and dependent on me, and I needed to help her. How could I be so mean to her? My mind completely turned, and I decided deep in my heart never to hurt her again.

When you and your daughter are sharing a close and happy moment, when she's not angry or upset, gently tell her that you're not going to be strict with her now that she's older. Tell her about impermanence, that we don't know how long a relationship between sisters or between mother and child will last. Impress upon her that we don't know whether our lives will be long or short, so during the time we have, we should be very loving and kind to one another.

You could also explain that she will have to face the consequences of her actions. The point isn't who is right or wrong, but that if she acts out of anger, those around her will respond in kind and everyone will suffer. She and the rest of the family will be miserable. Since our time together is so brief, why spoil it? Suggest how she could make better choices that might make everyone happier.

Talking to your daughter a few times like this when things are going well will bring you closer, and she may slowly change. Being inflexible and harsh will only create more problems. You don't have much choice, and there's really nothing to lose.

VINCENT: I feel more like a friend than a parent to my five-year-old son. Is that all right?

RINPOCHE: Being parents doesn't just mean being in touch with our children. It means thinking about how to benefit them and assessing what they will need from now until their death. Sometimes it also means being willing to do things that may upset them temporarily in order to prevent a negative habit from developing.

It's good to be friends with your child, but a friend usually focuses only on short-term fun and happiness. Your child needs you to be a parent—someone more mature, aware, and protective than a friend. It's your job to respond carefully to anything he does or says that might be harmful now or in the future.

IMANI: What can we do as single parents? We have full responsibility for our children; we have to do everything. It's difficult.

RINPOCHE: It is difficult, there's no getting around that. It's like trying to hold a hot clay pot—if you drop it, it will break, but if you don't, it will burn your hands. Do what you can—love your children in every way possible—and don't feel guilty about what you can't do. Be satisfied with what you're able to offer; you're doing your best.

8

Bringing People Together

IMANI: The spiritual truths you're talking about definitely aren't supported in the world I move in. I deal with many people who just don't operate with principles anywhere close to these. How can I uphold these teachings in my work environment?

RINPOCHE: When you return to work after attending this training, it is very important not to make a big deal out of what you have learned. Don't go back and insist that this is how things should be done. The more you push, the more others will resist. It is best to demonstrate these principles by example as you apply them to different situations.

Wherever you work—in a university or in a corporate, non-profit, religious, or other setting—the same interpersonal problems will arise, and the same approaches can help you solve them. No matter how much you try to live according to spiritual teachings, things won't always go smoothly. Some people will support what you are trying to do, but others won't like it, will misunderstand you, or even be hostile.

When you are criticized, consider whether what has been said is true. Maybe you really did make a mistake, or perhaps the critic is just having a bad day. By being open, you give space to a contentious co-worker, creating the potential for conflict resolution.

If somebody says something upsetting, instead of dwelling on it and asking why she said it, just drop it. Understand that if she is unhappy for some reason, anything may cause her to fly off the handle. When you let the situation go, there will be fewer hurt feelings all around.

When you prepare food for guests, you want to offer them your best. If they are happy, that's wonderful. But if they aren't, you don't think, "What's wrong with these people? Why don't they like my food?" Instead, you simply accept their differences in taste and attitude.

To act effectively, you need to be skillful. Seek your own best advice and be open to the counsel of others. Talk with those who have good heart, who understand and support the organization's goals. Check your motivation, and don't assume that your ideas and strategies are best.

If people disagree with you, always give them a chance to share their ideas, no matter how forcefully they may express them. Be patient. Don't give voice to your own disagreement, but skillfully offer some of your ideas with a clear and steady intention.

Don't think that, just because you're on the board of directors or have an impressive job title, everyone should operate according to your dictates. This is self-centered. Nor is it useful to sit back feeling that because you're such a peaceful, spiritual person with few strong attachments, you can let others do whatever they want. The people with the most helpful things to say in groups don't necessarily talk a lot; it is usually those with limited understanding, confusion, or largely selfish motivation who hold the floor. They may influence people who have good intentions but are unable to see the larger picture. If you don't communicate your point of view, the group's purpose might be lost or thwarted.

Some people's words or actions create a great deal of suffering for themselves and others. You can see that they are unhappy and will only bring more misery into their own lives and into your common pursuits. Always respond to them with pure heart, seeking to protect them from the effects of their confusion.

With this understanding, no matter how many problems arise, you will continue to work patiently and diligently, not for your own benefit, but for that of others. I'm not saying it's easy, but it is possible to have a positive impact.

IMANI: What should we do when the difference of opinion among decision makers makes it difficult to act?

RINPOCHE: When we work with others, it is most important for us to be accepting. On your board of directors, there might be a dozen people with a lot of experience and many different ideas. Each thinks he knows what is best based on his experience and temperament.

There are two ways to approach a group like this. You can listen, think about what you've heard, and evaluate each person's position. Or you can react, constantly objecting to other points of view. The first strategy, staying receptive, is much more effective because flexibility gives the group room to find some common ground. Don't stubbornly hold on to your own ideas to the bitter end, as if this were some sort of virtue in itself. Give up your attachment to what you have always thought was best. No matter how right you may think you are, trying to impose your opinion on others is wrong. Be open to the possibility of a better way of doing things. This will only create virtue and gain, and ultimately no loss.

You may think that a cup belongs here, but someone else may want to set it there. If it would make her happy, put the cup over there—you'll lose nothing by doing so. There is no benefit in being rigid and elaborating on all the reasons for your preference. If no real damage would result from letting her prevail, she'll feel better and you will have made more room to negotiate in the future on things that really matter.

Later, if some burning issue arises—one in which benefit or harm is truly at stake—you may choose to discuss it and persist. She will be more receptive to you because you will have already created a supportive, open environment. From your example, others will learn the same approach. Often the kind of impasse you describe can be resolved using such skillful means.

HELEN: How can we bring different business or political factions together?

RINPOCHE: With love and compassion, we have the greatest potential to bring people together harmoniously, no matter how organized they may be against one another's views. The extent to which we develop these qualities determines the degree to which we can benefit others in any circumstance. They have a magnetizing influence. A newborn baby reaches for his mother, not because he can differentiate her from other women, but because he responds to her love and compassion. We need to cultivate a similar ability to offer security and comfort. Then others will trust and respect us, and recognize in our attitude something they value.

Good heart is really the key, in both a spiritual and a worldly sense. These days, spiritual practitioners are sometimes weak in this regard. Many place their hopes on spiritual methods without doing the basic work of developing love and compassion, so they don't make much progress. The four immeasurable qualities— equanimity, compassion, love, and rejoicing—are truly the doors to happiness for ourselves and others, the best means for achieving conflict resolution, and the basis for authentic meditation.

DARYL: Sometimes it seems that the only way to bring people closer together is to expose underlying conflicts in order to resolve them. Is this true? Is it helpful to be up-front about our anger if we feel it's impeding conflict resolution?

RINPOCHE: There are two avenues to resolving conflict. First, those involved can try to correct their own minds and approaches, and these changes will then be reflected outwardly. Rather than insisting on their own way, they might work inwardly with their attachment so that, if necessary, they can concede to their co-workers without regret.

However, those who don't have the spiritual tools necessary to take this approach won't resolve anything by either repressing their feelings or angrily blurting out what they think is at issue. It is better if they talk to each other in a clear, truthful way. By calmly communicating the history of the problem and proposing a solution, they can facilitate mutual understanding.

Some people feel compelled to be completely honest and speak out at all times. But this doesn't usually work in mediation. In Tibetan culture, we don't bring dissenting parties together. They tend to be very emotional and to speak harshly, which only intensifies the problem. Instead, a mediator meets with each person individually. He makes sure that he understands each one's version of the conflict before interpreting it in a way the other party can hear. This way, emotions aren't stirred and the situation doesn't deteriorate.

There is a Tibetan saying about changing the words of a message to convey its meaning in a kinder way. Softening the original language isn't nonvirtuous, because the motivation isn't self-serving. Rather, it reflects the compassionate wish to bring people together. In this way, each party can consider the other's point of view, and a decision can be made based on understanding. The mediator plays a very active role.

TYLER: You said that in some instances of unresolved conflict, it's better to give in to the other person because in the long term you don't actually lose. So with an environmental issue like the clear-cutting of forests, where there are two distinct sides, does that mean compromising or giving the other side what would seem like a victory just to open up the possibility of a dialogue?

RINPOCHE: Though I don't have any experience in this matter, from what I've heard I feel that the case each side makes is understandable. If the two sides can speak to each other and get down to the underlying points of consensus, they might find room to negotiate. From there, they need to be willing to compromise; otherwise, neither side will achieve its goals.

A Tibetan adage says that when people suffer from lice, we can't blame the lice. They are hungry and have to eat. But neither can we blame the people who pinch and throw the lice away because they don't want their flesh eaten.

It's the same with environmentalists and the timber industry. We can't blame either side, nor is there any basic difference between them in terms of human interests. People in the timber industry want to keep their jobs. Environmentalists believe that we need to protect the environment for future generations. Without forests, there will be fewer resources, including jobs. Maybe this perspective could provide some common ground.

HELEN: What about when everyone means well, but all disagree about how something should be done?

RINPOCHE: As long as everyone has pure motivation, only virtue is created. There was once a man who made tsa-tsas, small clay representations of enlightened mind. He left them in many different places so that passers-by could receive their blessings. Another man saw one of the *tsa-tsas* by the side of the road and thought, "Someone put this tsa-tsa where the rain could destroy it. I'd better protect it." He covered it with the only thing he could find, the discarded sole of an old shoe. Yet another man came along and thought, "Covering a tsa-tsa with the sole of a shoe is disrespectful; I'd best remove it." So he took it off. Though their actions seemed opposed, each man had pure motivation and so made the same virtue.

Remembering everyone's basic intention will help you to appreciate rather than resent the efforts of others in your organization and to become more patient and skillful in your interactions.

HELEN: What do you do if the neuroses or habits of some of your co-workers are so counterproductive that accomplishing anything seems hopeless?

RINPOCHE: It's always best to try to rectify rather than give up on such a situation. Something can usually be done to achieve a peaceful resolution or to remedy some aspect of the problem, no matter how challenging it may seem.

Those with problems—not those without them—are the ones who need support. Some people can't change. But often, if you keep trying, you can help others to recognize their mistakes, to learn and benefit from the process. Patience is crucial because change won't happen immediately. If you do everything you can for someone and she turns against you, keep trying, again and again, in different ways. Slowly, you will see some change.

I have some experience in this area. I am very short-tempered, but when working with difficult people, I know that if I lose my patience, they won't keep theirs. As a teacher, if I lose my temper, how can I hope to help them?

In dealing with somebody's difficult behavior or attitude, I don't criticize or correct her right away, but rather try to reassure her. I say something like, "We're all human. We all make mistakes. This is fixable; don't worry about it." Then, gradually, I will try to solve the problem, either through example or indirectly, by talking to a group or someone else in her presence. Sometimes I can improve things with an act of generosity, other times with praise. Sometimes a display of wrath will help, but because that doesn't usually work, I explore other methods.

The Buddha said that there are four means of benefiting others. The first is generosity. We can offer a gift of our time as we listen and try to counsel. The second is praise. If we praise rather than criticize someone, she will relax and feel safer, more trusting, and receptive. The third is communication. Once this door is open, we can gently and slowly help others understand the nature of their problems and possible solutions. The fourth is action—demonstrating a solution with our conduct. To be of greatest benefit, we must use all four methods, whenever appropriate, to the best of our ability.

DARYL: When working in an activist group, how do we deal with people whose motivation isn't pure, who consciously or unconsciously disrupt the group with their personal agendas? How do we distinguish between those who would undermine us and those who are merely disruptive? If we can't prove negative intention, how do we deal with subversion?

RINPOCHE: Subversive intent is difficult to handle, of course. But it isn't as common in everyday organizational conflict as are problems arising from inexperience or ignorance. In either case, the principles of this training could be used to establish a set of commitments or guidelines that would serve as a basis for participation. They could include clearly delineated and agreed-upon standards of motivation and behavior. Such a framework could define how the group dealt with whatever arose, either internally or externally. Everything could be discussed and recorded in detail. Then each new participant would be required to uphold these commitments. A failure to do so could expose someone with ill intent. A basis would exist for determining if change or correction was necessary.

HELEN: This doesn't make sense to me, because it flies in the face of so many people's experience. Those infiltrating your group could pretend to subscribe to your principles and later do their best to destroy you. By the time you confronted them about not fulfilling their commitments, it might be too late. I guess what I'm looking for is a heart detector. Maybe we just have to know that we're open and vulnerable, and then do what we can.

RINPOCHE: Once, a very poor Tibetan woman on pilgrimage came to a sacred statue of the Buddha. All she had to offer was turnip soup. So she said, "Buddha, you may not like this, it may not be what you want, but it's all I have, so please accept my offering."

You can only do your best. At least it is worth your heartfelt effort. If each participant makes the same commitment, it won't be so easy to destroy the organization. Even if the problem becomes insurmountable, at least you've tried. Maybe your efforts will help. Maybe they won't.

Some people are cured by a doctor's medicine and some aren't. She still tries to assist them, still tries to do the best she can. Wherever you work, pure motivation will ensure that your efforts have a pure foundation. Beyond that, success cannot be guaranteed. That's up to karma.

9

Walking the Bodhisattva Path

WE BEGIN OUR JOURNEY on the bodhisattva path by checking our motivation for everything we do. Are we truly attempting to serve others, or are we only trying to benefit ourselves? We aren't enlightened; we do have selfish habits. But with diligent effort, we can change them. Practicing equanimity antidotes our pride and tendency to judge. Love antidotes anger, compassion antidotes desire, and rejoicing antidotes jealousy. Developing equal love, compassion, and rejoicing for all beings, and trying to repay their motherly kindness, results in better dreams for ourselves and others. Developing great equanimity through realization of the absolute truth purifies ignorance, so that we can begin to see through the dream, eventually awaken, and help others do the same.

Although these four immeasurable qualities are inherent within all of us, they are obscured by mind's poisons. As we purify those poisons, the four immeasurables are revealed to be the reflection of mind's nature and manifest effortlessly.

At the same time that we undertake our own practice, we make every effort to end the suffering of others. We aspire that each action of our body, speech, and mind contribute to the temporary and ultimate happiness of all beings. When we act with such motivation, we create incalculable benefit, for the extent of our virtue is determined by the scope of our motivation, not by that of the action itself.

When we do something to ease suffering without the specific intention of benefiting all beings without distinction, the virtue that results will infallibly produce happiness, but it will be impermanent. Virtue is inexhaustible only when we are motivated by bodhicitta. Even giving a few breadcrumbs to a hungry bird with the aspiration to produce temporary and ultimate benefit for all beings will create unending virtue.

Acting virtuously within the conceptual framework of relative truth, we are bound by the experience of self, immersed in the duality of self and other. Therefore, the virtue created is vulnerable to destruction by the effects of self-interest—mind's poisons—such as a feeling of self-worth for being useful, attachment to our way of helping, or aversion to another way. When no self-clinging is involved, the virtue cannot be destroyed.

However, even with our dualistic perspective, we can still protect and increase our virtue by always establishing pure motivation before we act and afterward dedicating the merit to the temporary and ultimate welfare of all beings. This way, the merit is sealed and cannot be destroyed. Otherwise, just as a single spark can set fire to an entire haystack, one moment of anger can incinerate great stores of virtue.

Merit that we have dedicated accumulates in the interest-bearing bodhisattva bank account. Just as money that we invest instead of squandering will multiply, producing more to enjoy and share, pure-hearted motivation and dedication will exponentially increase our ability to help others. Given the pervasive suffering in the world, helping several people in a day doesn't seem to have much impact. But if we dedicate to all beings the virtue of what we have done, the merit increases immeasurably. Like a raindrop blending inseparably with the ocean, the dedicated virtue of one or two kind acts merges with the ocean of merit created by buddhas and bodhisattvas and becomes a resource for all beings in all realms. Such indestructible merit never ceases to benefit, like a perennial that flowers year after year.

Accumulating and dedicating merit out of self-interest, on the other hand, will only produce temporary benefit. There was once a practitioner with a strong desire to sit on a throne like the high lamas. So he accumulated a lot of merit, offering butter lamps and food and practicing generosity. He didn't want to benefit anyone; he merely wanted prestige and recognition. His self-centered motivation and dedication led to rebirth as a rabbit that one day hopped into a monastery, right up onto a throne. Because he had accumulated so much merit, his wishes had a certain power, but not in the way he had intended. Moreover, all of his merit was exhausted in that single moment.

Merit purely dedicated by a group vastly increases the power of dedication of each individual in that group. At a certain monastery in Tibet, there lived a monk whom everyone liked. One day a fellow monk asked the head lama, "Why is he so likable? Is he a great bodhisattva?"

The lama replied, "No, he's no great bodhisattva. In his last life, he was a fat sheep. When the sheep died, the owners prepared the meat for a huge feast. All of the guests rejoiced and, at the end of the meal, dedicated the merit to the animal they had eaten. As a result, the sheep took rebirth as this well-liked monk."

We can dedicate on many levels. We might wish that, by our merit, the negative karma of all beings be purified and they find temporary and ultimate happiness. Or we might wish that all beings' mental poisons be eliminated so that no one will ever again create negative karma. Even more profoundly, we might wish that the poisons be transmuted and their pure essence revealed. Dedicating merit to the short-term welfare of all beings brings benefit only within the dream of samsara. Ultimate dedication involves the aspiration that all beings fully awaken from the dream.

There are two ways to dedicate merit. First, though we are not yet true bodhisattvas with stable realization of mind's nature, we can aspire that our dedication be like that of all buddhas and bodhisattvas. Second, if we have done enough spiritual practice, we can dedicate with the recognition of mind's nature; by this "great dedication," we accumulate wisdom.

To understand the accumulation of wisdom, consider an act of generosity, like giving someone an apple. Most of us believe unquestionably in the existence of the giver, the act of giving, and the recipient. These three aspects of subject, object, and the interaction between them are referred to as the three spheres. Though it seems real, the experience of giving is actually illusory or dreamlike. If we dream at night about offering someone an apple, the three spheres function in the context of the dream. But when we wake up, we realize that ultimately nothing happened; there was no apple, and no one giving or receiving it.

We have a deeply ingrained habit of believing that our everyday reality—this long dream we call life—is inherently true. This is ignorance. Because we don't recognize that we're dreaming, we have attachment or aversion to the different circumstances that arise. Attachment, aversion, and ignorance perpetuate the dream. As we dream, we create more dreams. Because our wisdom is obscured by confusion and mental poisons, we have little ability to help. However, by practicing the methods of the bodhisattva path, we can realize the true nature of this dream so that we are no longer lost in it. The eighty-four *mahasiddhas,* greatly accomplished bodhisattvas of Buddhist India, attained complete realization of the absolute truth and were so fully aware of the dreamlike quality of reality that they could leave footprints in solid rock and fly in the sky.

Through meditation, we too can awaken to the absolute truth and see through our experience, becoming masters of illusion. The great Shantideva said that mind's nature cannot be experienced with the intellect or grasped by ordinary concepts. Still, we need to begin somewhere, and words can be helpful. They are like a finger pointing to the moon, giving some indication of where to find it. But to have an actual experience of our true nature, we must meditate.

Water left in a bitter wind will freeze. It may seem as if the water has disappeared, replaced by ice. But the ice is not separate from the water; if we apply heat, the ice will melt and become fluid. The water is like the true nature of mind, absolute truth. The freezing wind is attachment and aversion, hope and fear, harmful thoughts and actions. The ice is our current experience of reality, relative truth. Meditation warms the chill of our obscurations so that mind's nature becomes apparent.

Because the foundation of our experience is the two truths, relative and absolute, to attain enlightenment we practice the two accumulations of merit and wisdom. Within our dream reality, we accumulate merit in order to benefit the dreamers. We simultaneously maintain recognition of the absolute truth of the dream, accumulating wisdom, in order to wake up. This is how we walk the bodhisattva path.

ORLIN: I don't understand how wisdom compels a bodhisattva to act instead of just sitting back and enjoying the dream.

RINPOCHE: A bodhisattva sees through appearances and realizes the empty, or dreamlike, nature of all phenomena. Just as an adult watching children build a sandcastle knows that what they are doing is only make-believe, a bodhisattva understands that all phenomena are illusory, like child's play. To a bodhisattva, everything that happens is like the magnificent appearance of a dream.

If during a night's dream we realize that we are dreaming, nothing that happens will have much effect on us. We can walk right up to a dream tiger and put our head in its mouth. Its hot breath won't disturb us because we know that we're dreaming. Similarly, it doesn't matter to a bodhisattva if someone wants her arm or leg, because she knows that she is offering a dream arm or a dream leg to a dream being in a dream world. This makes her fearless in her efforts to end suffering.

A bodhisattva understands with compassion that most beings don't realize the dreamlike nature of experience and, believing it to be true, become overpowered by it. When we don't know we're dreaming, our dreams are real for us. And within that reality, there is pain. A bodhisattva's wisdom gives rise to unceasing compassion and the fearless commitment to uproot the causes and conditions of all dreamers' misery.

TERESA: Are you saying that because we can make the dream of life anything we want, we have to be careful about what we choose—enlightenment, peace, or conflict?

RINPOCHE: That's it. Now we're in the midst of a dream. If it's a bad one, we can transform it by abandoning negative actions and embracing positive ones. But a good dream is still a dream. First, we need to improve this dream of life. Then we need to wake up, completely.

TERESA: Can we benefit even those who have harmed us or who don't want our help, just by dedicating merit?

RINPOCHE: In the grand scheme of things, we have a connection with all beings. Our relationships with others, positive or negative, are like links in a chain. So we pray that every being be liberated by our pure intentions, activities, and dedication. Whenever you dedicate merit, think of it as putting money in a savings account on behalf of all others.

In some cases, dedicating merit may be the only thing you can do on behalf of another. If you want to help someone in an abusive relationship, you have to be extremely skillful so as not to arouse anger, the desire to retaliate, or some other negative reaction in either person. If nothing else, you can pray for and dedicate merit to them.

It's as if all suffering beings inhabit a dark room illuminated by a single oil lamp. The virtuous thoughts and actions, and the dedication of merit, of anyone in the room add oil to the lamp. Everyone there benefits when the flame burns brighter and longer. Every harmful, negative thought or action consumes the oil, increasing the darkness.

The power to make change lies in our own hands, but we must be patient. Even if there is no immediate benefit, our efforts will not have been in vain. When we create and dedicate virtue unspoiled by anger or regret, the merit will eventually ripen for those we wish to help. By dedicating the merit to all beings, we add oil to the lamp that lights the way for everyone.

ALEXANDRA: How is our accumulated merit distributed to others? Why do some people seem to derive more benefit than others?

RINPOCHE: Though we have a connection to all beings, it is easier to help those with whom we are closely linked, especially if they are receptive.

A story illustrates the power of a close connection. When one member of a very wealthy family died, the family was anxious to find out where he had taken rebirth. After some time, a great lama passed through the area. The family asked him what had happened to their departed family member. Rather than answering the question directly, the lama suggested that they sponsor a reading of the Kangyur, the 108 volumes of the Buddha's teachings. The family erected big felt tents and invited thirty monks, who came and began to read the texts.

All this time, a local yogi knew that the deceased man had taken rebirth as a snake. As the texts were read, the yogi saw the snake suddenly crushed to death by a rockslide. Due to the virtue created by the family's sponsoring of the reading, combined with their close connection and dedication of merit to him, the snake was immediately reborn as a human.

It doesn't matter whether our connection is positive, as with someone we love and are trying to help, or negative, as with someone we've harmed intentionally or inadvertently. We prefer positive relationships, but negative ones are just as powerful. The connection between you and the chicken on your plate is one of suffering and death for the chicken, and one of good fortune for you. Nevertheless, its body is nourishing yours, so your prayers and dedication of merit will have a particularly strong impact.

HELEN: For months at a time, I can be tremendously active and capable of helping others. Inevitably, a difficult situation arises, and I despair of ever making any difference in the world whatsoever. I realize that good heart is the way to go, but how can I deal with these periods of burnout?

RINPOCHE: Ideally, we serve others with pure heart, not expecting gratitude, payment, or recognition. We accept complaints with equanimity and patiently continue, knowing that people don't always see the purpose of what we're doing. Though our actions may seem insignificant or unproductive, if our motivation is pure and we dedicate the merit expansively, we generate great virtue. Though we may not accomplish what we set out to do, auspicious conditions and our ability to benefit others in the future will only increase.

No effort is wasted; when someone witnesses our loving kindness, he sees a new way of responding to anger or aggression. This becomes a reference point in his mind that, like a seed, will eventually flower when conditions ripen. Then when we dedicate the virtue, our loving kindness will extend to all beings.

We mustn't become discouraged if someone we are trying to help continues to experience the results of her negative karma and, in the process, creates the causes for future suffering. Instead, because she doesn't have enough merit for her suffering to end, we must redouble our efforts to accumulate merit and dedicate it to her and others.

We're not out to accomplish selfish aims. We are trying to establish the causes of lasting happiness for all beings. By purifying our self-interest and mental poisons, we develop a heroic mind. The process of going beyond suffering and helping others do the same is the way of the bodhisattva.

ALEXANDRA: I hate to harp on this, but how do we ensure our own benefit while we're helping others?

RINPOCHE: If we do whatever we can to reach out, help, and serve others, our own merit will naturally increase and infallibly produce benefit for ourselves as well—infallibly.

∼

ANTIDOTING: WORKING WITH MIND'S POISONS

When we're involved in our daily lives, at home watching the news, or simply reflecting on the day's events, instead of focusing on the behavior of everyone else as though we were looking out a window, we watch our mind as if looking into a mirror:

• If we see judgment, pride, or bias, we practice one or more of the meditations on equanimity (pp. 43-46).

• If we see selfish attachment, grasping, or miserliness, we can antidote it with compassion (p. 87) and with the "Tonglen: Taking and Sending" meditation (p. 106).

• If we see anger, fear, or aversion, we can antidote it with one of the meditations for transforming anger (pp. 70-71), or we can practice the meditations on loving kindness (pp. 104-107).

• If we see jealousy and competitiveness, we rejoice in others' good fortune (p. 104).

• If we are confused and not sure what to do inwardly or outwardly, we can ask ourselves what would produce the most virtue and the least nonvirtue, in the short and long term, for everyone involved. We can review the teachings we've read or received, or, if we have a relationship to prayer, we can refresh our pure motivation (p. 26), antidote whatever poisons are present in our mind (p. 185), and pray that whatever is truly best in the short and long term, for all beings equally, become readily apparent. We can also remind ourselves that our experience, vivid though it may seem, is the mirage-like display of our mind. Observing every aspect of our outer and inner landscapes until we are convinced that they are illusory and dreamlike, we then let the mind rest.

Ideally, we do one or more of the above meditations until we can genuinely reestablish pure motivation, whether at home or in the world. Then we let the mind rest.

PART II

A Change of Course

10

The Roots of Happiness and Suffering

WHEREVER WE LIVE, whatever our color, culture, or religion, we all want to avoid suffering and find a stable source of contentment and fulfillment. Among the various realms of experience, the human realm offers the greatest opportunity for accomplishing this. As human beings, we are capable of bringing about change using our mind. Unlike animals, we have the ability to understand complex concepts. We can contemplate what we have heard or read, and validate or refute it. We can act on our beliefs, not with blind faith, but after extensive examination and analysis. Because of this, the human body and mind together constitute a unique and precious vehicle that can potentially take us completely beyond suffering in this very lifetime.

So why are we unable to avoid suffering or stabilize fleeting moments of happiness? The underlying problem is that we don't know what to abandon and what to accept in our quest for enduring happiness. Our self-oriented motivation leads us to act in ways that only produce more suffering and further obscure the true sources of contentment. We tend to focus on what we don't have—our catalogue of wants—and obsess over surmountable difficulties. This dissatisfaction blinds us to our inherent qualities, which we can otherwise use to benefit ourselves and others. It is as if in trying to improve our health, we mistakenly drink poison, get sick and die, come back to life the next day, take the same poison, get sick and die, repeating the process again and again. This is the predicament of all beings.

Happiness and sadness arise in quick succession. Although we think that they result from outer objects and circumstances, it is actually the mind's reactions that give rise to our experience. For example, some people love chili pepper; they feel that food not blessed by it is not worth eating. Others hate chili pepper; they feel that food seasoned with it has been ruined. Though the substance is the same, people's minds react to it in different ways.

And so it is with everything. Each person has her own experience of outer circumstances and empowers this view with judgments and opinions. One might consider a certain individual a perfect friend, reliable in any situation. Another might find the same individual completely untrustworthy. Again, it is their minds that regard the same person in different ways.

The ordinary mind assumes that everything perceived by the five senses is real, when ultimately none of it is. From this falsehood arises the interplay of separation and differentiation and, from that, hope, fear, attachment, aversion, pride, jealousy, and ignorance.

If we let the mind rest for a moment in a state of natural, uncontrived openness, all such emotion falls away. But then something comes to our attention. A curtain flutters, we hear a car or glimpse someone walking by. The mind immediately focuses on the stimulus as something outside of and other than the self. Making this distinction between self and other establishes the false perception we call duality. When we look at whatever has caught our attention and take note of details—its color, shape, size—we judge, evaluate, and further conceptualize. Then, on the basis of this assessment, we decide whether we like or dislike it. From our initial perception, these steps lead to full-blown attachment or aversion.

That is where our experience of suffering starts. If we want something and can't have it, we suffer. If we don't want something but it comes to us anyway, we suffer. We think our suffering is caused by the object we are attached or averse to, when actually the root can be found many steps earlier, in mind's dualistic perception.

This perception gives rise to the poisons of the mind, which produce hope and fear, actions and reactions—in short, the whole of samsaric experience. From duality arises the very idea of friend and enemy, which leads to conflicts between individuals, communities, and nations. Thus the ramifications of our misperception spin out into endless cycles of suffering.

Through our self-clinging, our complete identification with the concept of "I," we perpetuate samsara. All of us constantly seek ways to meet our own needs, thinking this will bring us happiness. Our existence is based on our obsessive desire to find fulfillment. Our hunger, like that of an addict, is all-consuming and insatiable, yet we succeed only in planting seeds of further misery. If instead we dedicate ourselves to meeting the needs of others, our selflessness, love, and compassion will become the medicine that cures us of our addiction and brings us to the state of perfect health called enlightenment.

All of our happiness and sorrow are the consequences of our past actions. Our experience is not accidental. If we scatter wheat seeds on the ground, they seem to disappear into the earth. But with proper conditions—sunshine, water, warmth—the seeds germinate and eventually become wheat. If we didn't know that they produced wheat, we might think that the cause and result were totally unconnected.

For lifetime after lifetime, in our waking state and in our dreams, we have reinforced the idea of self in our attempts to find fulfillment. But if self-centeredness produced happiness, we would all be enlightened by now. Focus on ourselves merely increases our attachment and aversion. Out of ignorance of what is harmful or beneficial to ourselves and others, we act upon our desire and anger, making one mistake after another. We have played out our ignorance, attachment, and aversion in so many ways for so many lifetimes that they seem a natural and inseparable part of us. Powerless in the face of the unending process of action and reaction and its consequences, we have no freedom. We may find some contentment, but once the karma supporting it becomes exhausted, the fruits of other negative actions ripen, happiness dissipates, and suffering arises in its place. This is true for every being.

People who want to bring about lasting peace need to clearly understand the goal, whether they think of themselves as spiritual practitioners or not. It doesn't matter what we call it; the goal is to end the suffering that abounds in the world. Though we may think that samsara is the problem, samsara is ultimately a state of mind. The key to ending suffering and finding peace lies in transforming our own mind—removing our negativity, enhancing our positive qualities, and revealing our true nature.

What obscures that nature is our identification with self. The "I" that so preoccupies us is not the essence of our being, but the very thing that prevents us from perceiving it. Just as the qualities of gold are not diminished by the ore in which it is embedded, our true nature is not diminished by our misunderstanding. Mind's nature will never change or cease; it has always been present within us. What remains after the smelting of gold ore is pure gold. Similarly, what remains after the process of refinement that we call the spiritual path is the fruition, our true nature fully revealed.

Four kinds of obscuration keep us from perceiving our nature. The first is intellectual obscuration, or duality—the belief that self, other, and everything that happens between them actually exist. The five poisons of the mind constitute the second. By following the push and pull of attachment and aversion, we create karma, the third. The fourth, habit, consists of the mental and emotional patterns established and reinforced by karma and mind's poisons, and carried over from one life to the next. If we remove these four obscurations, we will uproot the causes of suffering.

There are three basic kinds of suffering. The first is the suffering of change. Although we would like to be in control of every circumstance, this is impossible. Things change all the time. One day, we are ready for retirement; the next, we lose everything we own in the stock market and have to go back to work.

The second is suffering upon suffering. No matter how bad things are, they can always get worse. You are sick, and on top of that you wreck your car. Then the phone company turns your service off, even though you've paid the bill. There are no limits.

The third is pervasive suffering. Suffering permeates our experience like oil in a sesame seed. We don't see the oil until the seed is squeezed. Whenever we are squeezed by circumstances, the oil of suffering surfaces.

All beings in every realm suffer according to the degree and kind of delusion producing their reality. Whatever poisons predominate in their minds will determine the nature of their existence. Those whose minds are filled with virtue mixed with various poisons experience themselves as human beings. The minds of animals are characterized by mental dullness, their lives typified by suffering we can easily imagine or directly observe. Beings with stronger mental poisons inhabit realms of much greater misery that are difficult for us to even comprehend.

These realms cannot be located in space or proven to be true. Except for the human and animal realms, we cannot perceive them. Yet neither can we deny their existence, because to the beings who suffer, the experience is very real, just as the appearances of a nighttime dream seem real to us. Our dreams may unfold as nightmarish experiences of violence, but as soon as we wake up, we realize that nothing actually happened. They didn't ultimately exist, yet we cannot deny their vivid display. Nobody deliberately designed these torturous scenarios to make us suffer. They arose as projections of our mind, manifestations of anger.

If anger repeatedly fills the mind, it will eventually permeate our reality, and sooner or later we will experience what we call hell. In the same way, all the realms of samsara are manifestations of the mind's poisons and positive qualities.

A spiritually realized person perceives everything as a pureland, a reflection of mind's purity, whereas a being with extremely negative karma perceives his environment as hell. I have seen people in hospitals, screaming, "They're torturing me! They're burning me!" Although we don't share their experience, it is nevertheless their reality. Once, I met a woman who believed her hair was constantly catching on fire. Of course, I couldn't see the fire. Such people, whom we think of as insane, are tortured by the delusion of their mind.

If we put a toxic substance in the water supply, it will contaminate the water. Similarly, flooding the mind with a toxin such as hatred will alter our perception of reality. If a group of people share the same predominant mental poisons, they will experience the same reality.

During the time of the Buddha, a man from a different world system came to receive teachings from him. He commented to Shariputra, one of the Buddha's disciples, "How marvelous the Buddha's pureland is! What extraordinary qualities it has!"

Shariputra said, "There is nothing special about it. It's just an ordinary land, an ordinary place."

The man said, "No, no! It's an amazing pureland."

So they went to the Buddha to ask who was right. The Buddha replied, "It's true. This is my pureland. It has extraordinary qualities, but most people don't see them because of their obscurations."

I once knew an elderly monk who wore tattered clothes and was always hungry. In Tibet, if someone walks by your house, you invite him in and offer him food, because he has probably traveled a long way. At mealtime, this old monk could be found wandering by people's houses in the hope that they would give him something to eat. Whenever I traveled to perform a large ceremony, he would ask to come with me because the sponsors would be certain to make offerings to anyone in my party. During one of those ceremonies, he died.

Later, when we went to his home, we found that he had been sleeping on seven hundred silver coins. At that time in Tibet, a silver coin went a very long way. We were astonished, because we had always thought he was so poor.

Then someone noticed that one wall of the house looked different than the others. He knocked on it, joking that there was probably money inside. It sounded hollow, so we tore it down. We found several bags of silver coins, so heavy that two men could hardly lift one of them. Most of the people who had fed the monk were far poorer than he was.

Wealth and poverty are a state of mind. Someone may have a great deal of money and be a miserable, greedy person. Someone else may have very little and be content, even generous. Many people, wealthy and poor, think that their difficulties justify stealing or harming others. A person's lot in life doesn't indicate how much that person may suffer. People can live in palaces and still be desperate, lost, and lonely. Many wealthy people are unhappy about losing a hundred dollars, even if they still have a million. They are slaves to their money. The first thing they think about in the morning is making more, and the last thing they think about at night is how to avoid losing what they have.

The most severe suffering in the six realms—that of the hell realms—arises as a reflection of extreme hatred, anger, and cruelty. The increasingly unbearable heat of the eight hot hells, cold of the eight cold hells, and suffering of the neighboring hells creates unfathomable anguish. The bodies of hell-realm beings are as sensitive as our eyeballs. They endure torture for eons before their karma is exhausted, and they finally die, to be reborn in another realm. Listening to the teachings about hell causes us extreme discomfort, but just imagine what it's like for those suffering there.

The realm of hungry ghosts is characterized by starvation and thirst, unfulfilled need and desire. Whereas we would quickly die without water, hungry ghosts live on and on with an aching need for food and drink that they cannot possibly fulfill because of the limitations of their bodies and environment. The cause of such extreme deprivation is greed and miserliness.

The animal realm—a projection of ignorance and stupidity—is pervaded by the suffering of predation and domestication. Animals don't know from one second to the next whether they will become another being's meal. Many are beaten or tortured, used as the subjects of scientific experiments or as beasts of burden. Animals don't have the ability to transform the conditions that produce their suffering.

Rebirth in the three higher realms results from virtuous actions stained by mental poisons. Of the mixture of poisons that produce rebirth in the human realm, the most prominent is desire. Unable to get what we want or avoid what we do not, many of us have mental, physical, or emotional problems. Happiness and suffering fluctuate as our karma ripens and bears fruit. We all share the suffering of birth, sickness, old age, and death.

The jealous gods suffer from extreme competitiveness, covetousness, and continuous strife and warfare. Birth in this realm results from virtuous actions motivated by rivalry or jealousy, as when one helps others in order to prove one's own moral superiority.

The worldly god realm is extremely pleasurable, and a lifetime there lasts hundreds of thousands of our years. Because worldly gods never suffer, they have no incentive to change. The pride and self-interest mixed with virtue that lead to such an abundant and sensual existence blind them to its impermanence. Their fate is like that of a hot-air balloon that sooner or later cools and falls from the sky. Once their positive karma plays itself out, they begin the process of dying, which lasts for the equivalent of 350 human years. During that entire time, the worldly gods foresee the suffering they will experience in a lower realm. Because their merit has been depleted, they have no power to prevent this outcome. They have created neither the enormous amount of virtue necessary to remain in the god realm, nor the causes or conditions to be liberated from samsara. The suffering of their inevitable descent to a lower realm is like that of a fish thrown onto hot sand.

Clinging to bliss, clarity or stability in meditation can lead to a rebirth in a desire god realm, a form god realm, or a formless realm—a state of great bliss that can last for eons. In none of these realms can one attain liberation. As soon as one's karma is exhausted, as if waking from a night's sleep, one finds oneself back in a lower realm.

Although we in the human realm don't live as long as the gods or experience the same pleasure, we have a unique capacity to change and the potential to attain enlightenment. It is far easier and more effective to tame the mind and benefit others in this bittersweet human life.

One thing that keeps us from doing just that is false contentment. It is as if we are dangling off a precipitous cliff, holding on with one hand, yet thinking death is far away. The truth is that there is no time for complacency. If we lose our grip, our situation becomes hopeless.

We have to understand our potential as well as the cause of our predicament. If there were no real opportunity for change, there would be no reason for a spiritual path; our striving would be as futile as pressing sand to get sesame oil.

We now enjoy the very fortunate conditions of the human realm. We can find everything we need to develop and train the mind, and we have many occasions to practice patience, generosity, and compassion. So it is important that we apply ourselves well.

IMANI: Where does belief in God fit into your explanation of the cause of suffering? Are you saying that it's not God's will that we suffer?

RINPOCHE: Most people are sure that their suffering is someone else's fault. They often blame God or some other object of faith. But they are mistaken. No matter what our relationship to God or enlightened beings might be, they cannot create our happiness or eliminate our suffering. Masters from all traditions have gone to great lengths to try to benefit others, and there is no denying that they have helped suffering beings. Yet in spite of their extraordinary compassion and abilities, they haven't been able to eradicate suffering. They can teach us methods for producing happiness, but it's up to us to apply them. We are responsible for our own experience. Our mind's positive qualities give rise to positive circumstances. The mind's negativity gives rise to suffering. When we realize that our own mental poisons, arising from dualistic perception, are the root of the problem, we see that the key point is to transform the mind.

Our greatest mistake is that we don't recognize our intrinsic perfection. Our true nature is completely pure and unchanging—the absolute truth, whether you call it God, Buddha, or the nature of mind. But we are unable to perceive it. We don't realize that, in essence, everything is—and always has been—inherently perfect.

BEN: This may sound crazy, but if I'm already God, why should I worry about changing?

RINPOCHE: We need to change because we are unable to perceive the truth. We identify with the self and act out of self-interest, so we suffer.

TERESA: If I understand correctly, the god-realm rebirth you mentioned has nothing to do with our common notions of divinity.

RINPOCHE: There are two categories of gods. Deities known as wisdom beings are expressions of perfection. They are completely enlightened. Worldly gods, on the other hand, are imperfect, samsaric beings. They are very long-lived and powerful, but due to self-interest they remain trapped in samsara. One cannot attain enlightenment by relying on them.

TERESA: If we attain enlightenment, how do we help everyone still in samsara?

RINPOCHE: Enlightened beings are like the sun in the sky. The sun doesn't have to make an effort to shine, yet its light is reflected wherever there is a body of water. Reflections of enlightened mind arise effortlessly, spontaneously, wherever there is receptivity.

ALEXANDRA: How do you know if you are enlightened or getting there?

RINPOCHE: How do you know it is daytime? When all of your obscurations have been completely removed, wisdom dawns. It is clearly apparent. You couldn't mistake it.

A great practitioner can attain liberation in this lifetime. A less accomplished practitioner who is nevertheless very diligent will find several opportunities for liberation at the time of death.

HELEN: Most of us here aren't Buddhists, and we live and work with people who aren't Buddhists. How can we bring our understanding of the causes of happiness and suffering to our lives and work when those around us have a different way of seeing the world?

RINPOCHE: We all have different backgrounds and perspectives. We don't have to become Buddhists to work more effectively, but we do need to help people understand one another. Whatever we do, the underlying question is, Why are we doing it? If we are striving for peace, we act out of equal compassion for the victims of war as well as the war-makers. If we are animal rights activists, we act out of compassion not only for the animals being hurt or killed, but for those who harm them. In both cases, because the essence is compassion, the approach is spiritual.

If people who work hard to eliminate suffering aren't successful, they will continue to look for solutions. If they try one thing and it doesn't work, they will keep trying until something does. Because you are offering more comprehensive solutions, people will respond. Rather than picking all the poisonous fruit from a tree and throwing it on the ground, where it will eventually produce more poisonous trees, you are demonstrating means to uproot the tree altogether.

TERESA: Can prayer help end suffering?

RINPOCHE: The blessings of prayer help temporarily, but not ultimately. You can pray until your voice is gone and your throat is raw, but your prayers won't eliminate the fundamental cause of the problem you face. Each of us must address the confusion and delusion that we perpetuate with our own ordinary mind.

SARAH: Rinpoche, can we change an outward situation by perceiving it differently? If something negative happens to me or someone else, how can I act with compassion to transform the harm into benefit?

RINPOCHE: According to our karma, many different circumstances manifest in our lives. By meeting them with compassion, we don't necessarily change the circumstances themselves, but rather our experience of them.

HELEN: Battered women are often told that their situation isn't so bad, that others' suffering is worse. This discourages them from trying to find a solution.

RINPOCHE: One source of people's immediate suffering is their helplessness. When battered women come to you, affirm their ability to change things. Help them see that they have choices.

There are people and resources they can rely on for support. Their situation is quite different than that of someone with terminal cancer or someone in a war zone.

IMANI: In my limited understanding of Eastern spiritual traditions, I sense a more positive slant on things. But what I'm discovering in this training is a strong emphasis on suffering. I can listen to scary teachings about hell in church. How does one integrate the topic of suffering with other, more upbeat aspects of the teachings?

RINPOCHE: This brings up an extremely important point. It can be uncomfortable to contemplate the problems, confusion, and anguish of life; it's much easier to focus on peace and contentment. With so much reference to suffering in the media, we suffer simply from hearing about it. But once we acknowledge the extent and depth of pain in the world, we will naturally want to do whatever is necessary to help ourselves and others.

Many people fault Buddhism for its teachings on the misery not only of humans, but of all beings. Yet we need to know about suffering so that we can liberate ourselves and others. The Buddha taught that life is suffering, but he also taught that suffering has a cause, and if we eliminate that cause, suffering will come to an end.

If a sick person acknowledges her illness, she will go to a doctor and take the medicine he prescribes. If she ignores it, thinking it's not important or that she has no time to deal with it, she won't be able to take care of anyone or anything, much less herself, and her illness will only worsen.

There would be no point in thinking about the sickness if it were incurable. Similarly, pretending that there is no suffering will not liberate us. By looking suffering squarely in the face and finding its cause, we can gain freedom from it.

Suffering is one of the four topics that we contemplate in order to make the best of this life. Precious human birth, impermanence, karma, and suffering are known as the four thoughts that turn the mind. They are like special ingredients in a unique recipe for change; they will remove any obstacle and bring an unwavering quality to our spiritual practice. If we are prone to doom and gloom, lamenting that everything about our life is unacceptable, we can find encouragement by recognizing the preciousness of human life. Contemplating the impermanence of the objects of our desire will antidote our greed and grasping. If we are overwhelmed by misery, contemplating the suffering of others will help us realize our good fortune and develop compassion. When nothing makes sense, everything seems unjust, and we feel ineffective, we can remember karma.

On a more subtle level, thinking about impermanence relaxes our tendency to hold to the apparent truth of outer appearances. When we combine this contemplation with that of precious human birth, we'll understand the necessity of changing our priorities. Contemplating karma and the pervasiveness of suffering loosens our attachment to samsara.

When we contemplate the four thoughts, we start to see that much of what we do is based on wishful thinking. We begin to appreciate the urgency of our situation, and turn away from negative thoughts and actions, just as we would avoid a harmful diet when we are sick. Like putting gas in a car to make it run, contemplating the four thoughts will fuel our enthusiasm for the spiritual path. It will counteract our false contentment, laziness, and procrastination. It will also help us to clarify our goal, for it will become evident that any short-term benefit is unreliable and that, to benefit all beings ceaselessly, we must thoroughly uproot the causes of suffering in our own mind and in others'.

Samsara is a state of perpetual suffering; enlightenment is a state beyond suffering. Yet they are not so far apart. Whether we experience one or the other depends on whether we know the truth of our reality. We come to recognize that truth through meditation.

Meditation is not a matter of resting in a void, staving off concepts. It can help us develop both a deeper conceptual understanding of spiritual truths—such as the four thoughts—and nondual wisdom. Genuine meditation gives rise to a knowing quality that will make our work more effective and more beneficial.

~

CONTEMPLATING SUFFERING

Whether at home or in daily life, as we encounter suffering, we begin this meditation by asking ourselves if we can think of anyone throughout time and space who is beyond suffering, who has known happiness that is not fleeting. Then we let the mind rest.

Reflecting on our own lives, we examine whether we believe that the cause of our suffering lies in our self-centered habits and the poisons of the mind. Even if we are happy now, are we sowing seeds of future misery? Have we already planted seeds that haven't yet borne fruit? We contemplate these things again and again from different angles, thinking of different experiences in our lives. Then we rest the mind.

We give rise to compassion for the countless beings caught in the web of suffering with no understanding of its causes or the means to end it, and then let the mind rest.

We make a commitment to do whatever we can to free them from the causes and conditions of suffering, and then let the mind rest.

HOW SUFFERING BEGINS

To understand how suffering begins, we let the mind rest naturally, dropping all thoughts of past or future. What we find is openness without grasping, confusion, or suffering. The mind is aware and clear. Then we see or hear something and our awareness darts to it, like an arrow. Do we experience any tension, anxiety, or suffering in the act of perception itself?

Next, we may notice details—a shape, color, or volume. Do we experience any suffering at this point? Can our mind remain relaxed as we perceive these details? Do we immediately begin to assess, categorize, and judge?

If so, we then notice the sequence of our mental events. We either like what we see or we don't. Watching carefully, we can determine when disturbance first arises in our mind. Does liking the object lead to attachment? Do we think, "I need that"? Are we thinking that, if we don't get it, we will suffer? Does our not liking it make us want to get rid of it? If we can't avoid it, do we think we will suffer? Do we want to act on the basis of such feelings? Would our actions harm or benefit ourselves or others? Would they bring temporary and/or ultimate benefit?

It can be very instructive to watch, during our daily lives, how frequently we are self-absorbed. For example, while trying to help others—if we're really honest with ourselves—we'll likely notice the pervasiveness of more subtle and less conscious responses such as liking or disliking someone else's approach to helping, or wanting things to go differently, or being attached or averse to the way events are unfolding.

Recognizing the sequence as our mind moves from a peaceful state of rest to perception, judgment, and the appearance of emotional poisons and actions arising from these poisons, we can see the genesis in our mind of the four obscurations: duality, mental poisons, karma, and habitual patterns. We observe the process by which the relaxed state becomes disrupted, not by outer circumstances but by our mind's response to them. Over time, with practice, this perspective will become more natural and permeate our daily life, increasingly informing our conscious and unconscious choices and the actions of body and speech that follow those mental and emotional states.

11

Mind and Meditation

THE ROOT OF ALL DIFFICULTY and conflict lies in the mind; therefore, the solution to all difficulty and conflict lies in changing the mind. To do this, we practice meditation.

What is this mind that gives rise to the experience of happiness or suffering, to the ability to help or harm? When we search for it, we discover that it has no substance. It is joined with the physical body through karma, producing the experience of birth, aging, and death. But this process takes place in the body, not the mind; the body is like a shell in which the mind dwells. The mind, with its habit of embodiment, creates both dream and waking bodies. After death, freed from the physical body, it inhabits a mental body in the intermediate state, then another body in our next lifetime. Mind itself is beyond birth and death—it is a continuum. It is not born; it does not age or die.

If we try to describe mind, we discover that it has no color, shape, or size. If we try to locate it, we can find no place where it abides. So we cannot say that mind exists, because it escapes our rational investigation. Yet we cannot say that it does not exist, because it is the very source of these observations as well as of our entire experience of reality. In this way, it becomes apparent that our limited intellect simply cannot fathom the mind.

The ordinary mind, filled with positive and negative thoughts and emotions, constantly changes. It lacks freedom, for it is continuously influenced by external phenomena. Depending on our circumstances, we are happy, sad, up, down. If we received a penny for every thought that arose in the mind, the wealthiest person in the world would seem poor by comparison. Yet if we examine the stream of thought, we won't find any place where it dwells. The space between one thought and the next—and ultimately the essence of thought itself—is timeless and insubstantial.

Just as the sky is unchanged by rainbows, clouds, or lightning, the true nature of mind remains unaffected by the fluctuations of ordinary mind. Mind's nature is the foundation of the unceasing thoughts and emotions of the conceptual mind, just as the ocean is the source of the constant movement of waves arising and subsiding. In the same way that waves arise from the ocean yet are not separate from it, the ordinary mind is not separate from its nature.

Our true nature is always present. But the dualistic mind, like a show-off, takes the stage and steals the scene, making a great display of its needs and wants, attachments and aversions. Like ink in water, these poisons obscure our true nature, though it never actually changes. Thus the ordinary mind, through the filter of our poisons, projects a vast array of illusory appearances that arise inseparably from mind itself.

The true nature of the whole drama of subject-object experience lies beyond extremes. We cannot say that we are all one; if that were true, when one person found happiness, we would all be happy, or when one of us attained enlightenment, we would all become enlightened. Nor can we affirm that everything is separate and distinct, because the seemingly individual components of our experience are not ultimately true or existent; they are of one taste in their absolute nature.

Unaware of mind's nature, we are influenced by hopes and fears, absorbed in an unending stream of concepts. As if mistaking a chunk of gold for ordinary rock, we needlessly suffer from a sense of impoverishment. Although efforts to create happiness and end suffering are beneficial, only resting in the nature of mind will produce awakening. Knowing that recurring nightmares are only dreams doesn't relieve our nightly torment. Good dreams are better than incessant nightmares, but they still fall short of full realization of our true nature.

So our first step is to thoroughly examine and begin to uproot the causes of suffering. Seeing the predicament of beings, whether they are in pain at the moment or sowing the seeds of future misery, our love and compassion naturally increase. This leads to a firm commitment to train our mind through meditation, so that we can fully reveal its true nature and free others from delusion.

MEDITATION

The mind is like a television's remote control. If we know how to change channels, we can change the picture. Cyclic existence— from birth to death, to the intermediate state, and then to birth again—goes on continuously for every being. We have short and long lives, happy and sad ones. Throughout all of them, mind's true nature never changes. Yet its essential purity and our failure to recognize it exist simultaneously, just as the impurities in gold ore exist simultaneously with the gold. If we identify with the seeming truth of the ore, we find ourselves in this dream of samsara. By refining the ore, we reveal the gold, our true nature. We do that through meditation—training the mind, bringing it back repeatedly to a state of virtue or relaxation. With diligent practice, we can reveal our inherent wisdom. This is the only way to break free of the viselike grip of ignorance, which gives rise to all obscurations and ultimately all suffering. The Tibetan word for wisdom is *yeshe*. *Ye* means "timeless, pristine, primordial." *She* means "knowing"—knowing mind's true nature.

This wisdom does not usually come suddenly or quickly, however. Step by step, we gain a greater understanding of absolute truth. First, we listen with an open mind to spiritual teachings, to new ideas. At this point, more than acquiring "knowing," we are removing "not knowing." After hearing the teachings again and again, we develop a new perspective. This is called the wisdom that comes from listening to the teachings.

But this is only the beginning. We then use our intellect to ponder what we have learned. We identify our doubts, ask questions, and reflect on the answers. If we don't go through this process, trying to meditate is like attempting to sew with a two-pointed needle. But once we make the effort, we will be entirely clear as to why and how to meditate. Then we can meditate one-pointedly. Extensive reflection gives rise to what is called the wisdom that comes from contemplating the teachings. It resolves doubts, removes ignorance, and diminishes confusion.

However, we need to go further. It is possible to forget what we have contemplated unless we fully integrate our theoretical understanding into our mind and heart. The insight we gain while sitting on our meditation cushion can be difficult to access when we are in rush hour traffic or in situations of conflict. That process of assimilation happens through meditation.

We can understand intellectually that ignorance, attachment, and aversion prevent us from perceiving our intrinsic perfection. But mere understanding will not produce the direct realization of that perfection. If we just listen to teachings and think about our true nature but fail to meditate, we will never actually experience it. And we will remain as attached, ignorant, and angry as ever.

Through meditation, we counteract old habits. The tightly rolled paper that we take out of the closet after many years gradually assumes its natural state whether we roll it backward, place big rocks on the corners, or iron it flat. What we have heard becomes more obvious to us, and we develop a genuine experience of the truth of the teachings. This increases our faith and diligence, which in turn makes us want to practice even more, which further increases our faith and diligence, and so on.

This threefold process of exposure to the teachings, contemplation, and meditation enables us to transform negativity, awaken wisdom, and reveal mind's positive qualities. Then when difficult situations arise in our efforts to serve others, we will be prepared to act appropriately.

Remaining in a state of relaxation, free of thought, can be difficult for beginners. If we hold the mind too tightly, we will merely upset it, like a wild horse we try to tame by restraining it with a short tether. It will only rear up or pull away. We are not attempting to suppress mind's knowing quality. Instead, we allow the mind to use its natural function of conceptualization to engage in positive thought, just as if we built a large corral within which the horse could run freely. The mind experiences itself as free, yet runs within the corral of virtue.

Most people think that meditation just involves allowing the mind to rest in a nonconceptual state. But if we simply strive to let the mind relax without having applied methods to transform our habitual patterns, we won't see much change. If we push the "pause" button on a tape recorder, the sound will stop; when we release the button, the tape will continue to play the same tune. Just because we pause and take a break from our mental habits during resting meditation, this doesn't mean that we have erased the tape of habitual mind. To actually do so and record a new one, we don't force a nonconceptual state but instead engage in effortful meditation—repeatedly bringing the mind back to a spiritual topic or point of concentration, no matter how often we become distracted.

The method of effortful meditation that we use in the Bodhisattva Peace Training is contemplation. We repeatedly contemplate the teachings, imprinting them on the tape of the mind. Then when we press the pause button, relax, and release it, what we hear will be different than before. Contemplation has the power to change the mind's patterns, replacing our negative habits with virtuous thoughts.

We contemplate the teachings in light of our own experience hundreds of times throughout the day, whatever we are doing: walking, talking, eating. Instead of indulging in counterproductive meditation—focusing repetitively on self-centered thoughts that increase rather than reduce suffering—we reflect again and again on how we can best be of service. Or we contemplate how we unwittingly perpetuate the causes of suffering for ourselves and others.

Another way to contemplate is to imagine challenging situations and practice responding to them. For example, we might imagine a disagreement with someone. We could consider the short- and long-term consequences of following our impulse to be nasty. How would we generate love or compassion instead? Or we could contemplate how our knowledge of karma or suffering might alter our response.

Effortful meditation will produce a degree of understanding and some change in mind's habits but will not, by itself, bring enlightenment. Only effortless meditation—resting in recognition of mind's nature—will do that. Because the verb "to meditate" implies effort, in this training we use the phrase "allow the mind to rest or relax." Effortless meditation does not involve any striving; the mind simply abides in a state of relaxation that allows us to know its nature.

The ultimate point of effortless meditation is to recognize what is already there. We don't increase or improve the nature of mind by meditating, nor do we reduce or defile it by not meditating. If we could change mind's nature, it would necessarily be contrived and impermanent. But this is true only of ordinary mind.

The concepts and assumptions of ordinary mind mask its true nature. When we stop engaging our emotions and thoughts of past and future, they naturally subside. By resting in a state of openness, we allow the mind to become calm and stable so that we can taste its true nature, not intellectually, but as a direct experience.

At first, the state of rest won't last very long. Thoughts will arise. Instead of letting them run rampant, we direct them toward a spiritual topic, like compassion, karma, suffering, or equanimity. When the contemplation becomes stale, we drop it and let the mind relax again. We don't do anything special—we just let the busyness go. Once again, when thoughts arise, rather than suppress them, we direct them toward contemplation. We use one concept to antidote another. To antidote mind's habitual conceptualizing altogether, we allow the mind to rest.

In meditation, we work toward a balance between contemplation and mind at rest. Contemplating without resting is like stirring the sediment in a pond. On the other hand, resting without contemplating is like practicing archery without a target. We cut through mental dullness and attachment to emptiness through contemplation. Then we cut our attachment to concepts by letting the mind rest. We go back and forth, so that we are neither consumed by swirling concepts nor lost in a dull or comalike state free of thought.

The Buddha once had a student who told him he couldn't meditate. The Buddha asked, "What is your work?"

"I'm a musician," the student replied. "I play a stringed instrument."

The Buddha asked, "Is the sound of your instrument sweet if the strings are tight?"

"No."

"Is it sweet if the strings are too loose?"

"No."

"So what do you do?"

"I find a balance."

"That's how to meditate."

Alternating between contemplation and relaxation keeps the mind fresh, more wakeful. Effective meditation lies in the turn from one experience to the next, the point where the mind is instantly open and unadorned. Ideally, the mind in meditation is like water tumbling down a cliff. It becomes clearer each time it hits a rock and changes direction, until it reaches the bottom and is pure.

If we try exclusively to relax the mind for a long time, all kinds of concepts and distortions or stagnation can creep in. Therefore, in beginning meditation, it's best to devote ninety percent or more of our practice time to contemplating and ten percent or less to letting the mind rest. As our practice matures, the mind will remain alert and in a state of rest that is truly fresh for longer periods.

If we don't alternate between effortful and effortless meditation, we may become attached to temporary meditative experiences, such as bliss, clarity, or stability. These are natural by-products of meditation, just as smoke and sparks are by-products of fire. They are not the goal. The trick is not to become enamored of or lost in them. They can indeed eventually become opportunities to free ourselves from attachment rather than to indulge in it. But whether we have seemingly exalted experiences, such as visions of buddhas and bodhisattvas, or frightening, possibly painful mental or physical experiences, the point is not to get sidetracked, but to keep going, remaining consistent in our practice. Fascination with them will only take us off course and delay our realization of mind's true nature.

Through contemplation, we acquire greater understanding and compassion, and accumulate merit. By resting in mind's nature, we accumulate wisdom. These two accumulations lead to full actualization of the two facets of enlightened mind: nondual realization of the ultimate truth, and knowledge of all causes and conditions of past, present, and future.

In fact, these two methods are not so different. Both point the mind in a new direction, away from its ordinary habits.

Meditation also includes the periods between formal practice sessions when we maintain awareness of the illusory nature of our experience. We practice recognizing that neither our daytime reality (in which our night dreams don't intrude) nor our night dreams (in which our daytime reality is imperceptible) are inherently true. They are equally illusory. With compassion for beings, we regard whatever arises—positive or negative—as a dream, a mirage, a rainbow, a reflection of the moon in water, a phantom city, or a hallucination, and abide in equipoise.

In the beginning, hope and fear permeate our practice: we hope that we have found mind's nature or fear that we have not. But slowly, a seamless experience emerges that is beyond concepts of meditation and nonmeditation, beyond hope and fear, and we rest effortlessly, awake in the nature of mind.

PRAYER

Prayer is a way of creating intimacy between ourselves and enlightened beings. It doesn't matter what religion we follow. Even if we don't adhere to any particular tradition, we can still supplicate: "Whoever has enlightened qualities, please hear my prayer!"

Due to the pervasive presence of hope and fear in the mind, we place hope on those we think can help us, and fear those we think might harm us. In a spiritual context, we hope that an enlightened being, someone outside ourselves, will aid us by the power of that being's positive qualities.

However, the purpose of prayer is not to please enlightened beings so that they will grant our requests, like adults giving candy to well-behaved children. Rather, we pray in order to become receptive to their blessings, which are unconditional.

The loving kindness of wisdom beings is all-pervasive, yet as beginning practitioners we are like an impenetrable iron ball with no ring to catch the hook of their compassion. Even though our true nature is no different from that of wisdom beings, theirs, like gold, is fully apparent; ours, like gold ore, remains obscured. So we pray that our impenetrability will dissolve, that we may open to enlightened beings' limitless blessings, that our mental poisons will diminish and our qualities and ability to help others will increase. Eventually, as our practice of prayer deepens, the apparent separation between ourselves and those we supplicate will dissolve, and our inherent wisdom will dawn.

We pray not just for ourselves and those close to us, but for all beings, including our adversaries: "By your blessings, may I and all others overcome suffering and gain happiness now and ultimately." Such selflessness exponentially increases the power of our supplications. The more we pray, the more blessings we will receive. And the accumulation of prayers offered in the past will support us any time we pray.

Although it is helpful to pray when obstacles arise, we shouldn't do so with aversion to them or with attachment to what we want, because we cannot be certain that something is truly an obstacle. We are not omniscient.

Once, a Tibetan woman was traveling by airplane. The plane made a stop, and she got off to look around. Unfamiliar with the language and the airport, she missed her connecting flight, which crashed soon after takeoff. A prayer like "Don't let me miss this plane" as she ran to make the flight would have been sorely misguided.

We might pray to be spared a serious illness, yet that sickness could purify our karma or prevent something worse from happening were we to go on with life as usual. Because we don't know all the factors involved, we should always pray for whatever is truly best.

Prayer is an aspect of effortful meditation that we alternate with relaxation. Though we start with the dualistic concept that we are separate from perfection, we open our heart through prayer and devotion until we experience a falling away of that fictitious boundary. Once our heart has blended with the experience of perfection, we allow the mind to rest.

TYLER: You said it's not enough to listen to the teachings—we need to meditate. But what if we're looking for more information and understanding, and want to keep learning?

RINPOCHE: Aspiring to know more is wonderful, but first we must fully apply what we've already learned. We don't want to be like a hungry yak, always looking for the next clump of grass even as he eats the one in front of him. We should digest what we have received before going on to the next teaching. If we don't thoroughly contemplate and meditate, our understanding won't stick and we won't change much.

A *yeti* (a large, apelike animal) sitting at the mouth of a prairie-dog hole may think he's hit the jackpot. He reaches in, grabs a prairie dog, and, not satisfied with only one, sits on it while he reaches in to grab another. But as he leans forward, the first one runs away. He then sits on the second one; thinking he now has two, he reaches for a third. And so on.

In the same way, if we merely tuck the teachings away without contemplating them, we'll forget them. Then, when difficulties arise, we'll find them hard to apply because we never really assimilated them. We may understand the need for patience, for example, but the minute someone says something unkind, we lose our temper.

TERESA: When I contemplate compassion, I feel a lot of pain. When I let my mind rest, I feel joy; but as I experience that open space of the mind, I also feel fear. Am I doing something wrong?

RINPOCHE: The pain and fear are similar, in that both of them cause you to back off from your experience. As you stand at the edge of the precipice, you have to ask yourself, "Who is stuck here? Where is this feeling coming from?"

If you examine your fear or pain without reacting to it, you will see that it has no solid basis; it is as dreamlike as everything else. This frees your mind a little from the belief that it is real in the absolute sense.

All of us get stuck at some point in contemplation or meditation. If our experience is blissful, we become caught by our attachment, as if by the jaws of a crocodile. Just as easily, we can be gripped by fear. But rather than grasping with attachment or quaking with fear, we need to relax. Then we can begin to see through the concepts that play across the screen of the mind.

Deep understanding requires extensive contemplation, but by itself, such examination cannot unravel the tangled net of hope and fear. Only through the profound relaxation in which we recognize their true nature can these emotions be freed. When we indulge in mind's poisons, we only create knots of further obscuration. But just as we have tied these knots, we can untie them.

TYLER: I don't understand how not to lapse into dualism when I observe something happen.

RINPOCHE: A grandmother watching children play doesn't get caught up in their drama the way the children do. She doesn't grasp at or reject it; to her, it is simply play. We, on the other hand, invest appearances with a reality they don't have and get totally lost in them. However, with proper training, it is possible to neither become involved in a situation nor reject it, but to recognize it as play. We can simply allow it to arise and subside. Even as it occurs, it ceases, and so doesn't require our involvement or rejection.

Nondual awareness of the true nature of mind and phenomena is called "view." Effortless meditation involves neither grasping at nor rejecting appearances, but simply remaining in that relaxed space of mind, allowing them to resolve. The Buddhist tradition offers extremely profound teachings on this subject, but in essence the practice comes down to just this.

It isn't so difficult to understand these words conceptually, but they aren't easy to put into practice, because something always seduces us. Before we know it, we have lost the state of utter relaxation, and our ordinary mind has slipped into involvement or rejection.

Effortless meditation is difficult. It requires mature spiritual practice, which we develop through effortful meditation. This ripens the mind so that it can perceive what is otherwise imperceptible.

I am in my sixties, and although I use the same method, each year my meditation changes. It continues to deepen, to become more subtle, clear, and profound.

TYLER: So could you sum it up by saying that our thoughts and emotions are impermanent but the nature of mind is permanent?

RINPOCHE: There are two aspects of mind—mind as it is and mind as it acts or functions. The functioning aspect of the mind includes thought, which arises like a rainbow from a crystal. Concepts come and go, products of certain conditions, like the rainbow. If you take the crystal away, there is no rainbow. The nature of mind is the basis of all appearance; yet that nature itself does not change.

In one way, you could say that thoughts are impermanent, susceptible to outer conditions. On the other hand, they are empty, ultimately beyond concepts of permanence and impermanence.

TYLER: Is it better to meditate with our eyes open or closed? I've tried to meditate with my eyes open, but it's been tough. Can't I just close them and get some meditative ground under me first?

RINPOCHE: It is better to keep your eyes open. Phenomena are not the obstacle; grasping at them is. Grandparents don't have to close their eyes to feel calm as their grandchildren play. In meditation, we leave our senses open and equally balanced. Rather than accentuating vision, hearing, or feeling, we maintain an all-encompassing perception. Balance and openness are closer to nondual awareness. That awareness isn't dark, closed, or restricted. We don't need to shut anything out.

IMANI: What takes place in the mind of an older person who can't remember anything? If the mind is everlasting and constant, what about my mother, who appears to have lost her mind?

RINPOCHE: You're referring to mental faculties, not the nature of mind. The mind itself has no substance, but is joined with the physical body and a subtle body, which consists of subtle channels and energies. When the physical body is not sound, when it is sick or old, our mental faculties can become impaired. The ordinary mind becomes very dull, or irrational emotions arise. But mind's nature doesn't change. For example, even if a stroke causes paralysis and hinders one's speech or thought, that nature remains unchanged.

On the other hand, when the physical body is strong and the subtle energies flow smoothly, we have greater mental acuity. In meditation, we use specific postures to keep the subtle channels straight, so that these energies can move freely. This enhances our mental faculties.

ALEXANDRA: You mentioned something about the space between thoughts, the nature of mind having a timeless quality. Would that mean that an intuitive flash breaks the space-time barrier? When you suddenly have an insight or see something in the future, does that mean your mind is messing with time a little bit?

RINPOCHE: Nothing is messing and nothing is missing. It just implies a thinning of our obscurations, allowing the mind to reach beyond ordinary parameters.

There is an old story from India about a man who asked his friend, a powerful magician, to conjure up an illusion so that he could experience the dreamlike nature of phenomena. The magician smiled, poured his friend a cup of tea, and said, "Not today. Maybe some other time."

Before the man drank his tea, he went outside to find more wood for the fire and somehow lost his way in the forest. Night fell, and he grew very cold and hungry. The more he wandered in the dark, the more lost he became. As the sun rose, he came at last to a town that was completely unfamiliar to him. He had no money, so after a time began to beg, struggling day after day to survive.

He then wandered to another town, where eventually he found work, fell in love, married, and had a child. The child died just after birth, and he and his wife suffered tremendously. They had another baby who also died. Tragedy upon tragedy befell him. Still, the man worked very hard and built a home. Finally the couple had a third baby. That one survived for a while and brought them great happiness, but then died as well. At that point, they were no longer able to have children. Life became more difficult as they aged, until finally the man's wife died, and he was once again alone. So old that he could hardly move and nearly blind, he reflected on the passing of his life, feeling great sadness because his few moments of happiness had been so fleeting.

With that, the magician snapped his fingers and the man woke up. He asked the magician, "Why did you do that? I suffered so much and for so long."

The magician replied, "It wasn't all that long. Your tea isn't even cold."

We superimpose our concepts of time and space, like a grid, on our sense of reality, believing them to be valid units of measure. But when we begin to realize the truth of our experience, we see how arbitrary they really are.

VINCENT: At times, the methods you've taught us work for me, but usually my mind is wild—all over the place—and I feel that my meditation isn't cutting it at all.

RINPOCHE: Sometimes meditation seems hopeless, and we feel discouraged by the many negative thoughts that crowd the mind. We may even feel that they've actually increased since we started meditating. But that's not the case; they've been there all along. It's just that now we're noticing them, perhaps for the first time. This means that we're making progress. Our negativity shouldn't surprise us. After all, if we were perfect, there would be no reason to meditate. So as we watch the mind, when we see negative thoughts and emotions arise, rather than following them, we can let them go without giving them any power.

When we get discouraged, it helps to look back and observe how we've changed. If we are very diligent, we'll notice change every day—if not daily, then monthly, or at least over the course of a year. That will give us the impetus to go forward. In beginning practice, we may notice that positive, kind, and selfless thoughts arise only ten percent of the time. But the more we practice, such thoughts arise fifteen, twenty, or twenty-five percent of the time. We start to change.

TERESA: Should I contemplate while engaged in activity or only when I'm not doing anything else?

RINPOCHE: Try to apply contemplation to your activity. If you are watching the evening news, contemplate suffering. Or when you upset someone, contemplate karma. Then when you allow the mind to rest, remain aware. If you are sewing, let the mind settle with each stitch. Don't let it go here and there, following your thoughts. If you are writing, let the mind settle with the movement of the pen or your fingers on the keyboard. When the mind is aware, when it becomes one with your activity, you are protected from negative thinking. Maintaining awareness has the same effect as directing the mind toward positive thoughts, and it brings forth mind's positive qualities.

Centuries ago, the Indian mahasiddhas attained enlightenment while working at ordinary jobs. Some meditated while they pounded sesame seeds, others while they played musical instruments, dug ditches, or wove fabric. Regardless of what we do outwardly, bringing awareness to all our activities is meditation.

It's not enough to do an hour or two of formal meditation in the morning and let the mind run wild the rest of the day. In a tug of war, if two people are pitted against twenty-two, who is going to win? We need to practice as much as we can, contemplating or relaxing for short periods, many times throughout the day. Whenever we realize we've forgotten to do so, we bring the mind back.

TERESA: When I'm involved in different activities, I tend to become so absorbed that I forget to meditate. What can I do to remember?

RINPOCHE: Actually, you are meditating all day, but on the wrong things—things that will increase rather than reduce suffering. A hundred thousand times each day, we repeat the mantras "I," "me," "mine," "This is what I need," "This is what I want." This becomes our meditation.

Instead, establish a routine to remind yourself of others' needs, just as you would tie a string around your finger as a reminder to pick something up at the market. When you start your car, reestablish pure motivation, or as you pass others on the street, cultivate loving kindness. Meditation involves bringing something to mind, or the mind to something, again and again. If we think of compassion only during the one week of the year that we go on retreat or vacation, we will never fully develop it.

Once there was a respected lama whose mother had very negative habits. He begged her to meditate to purify her karma, but she wasn't at all interested. So he placed some bells on the spindle of her spinning wheel, on the door to her room, and on her kitchen utensils. He then requested, "Mother, please, whenever you hear a bell ring, repeat the mantra *Om Mani Padme Hung.*" The old woman truly loved her son and wanted to make him happy, so whenever she heard one of the bells ring, she would say, "*Tah Om Mani Padme Hung,*" which was like repeating, "I'm obligated to pay this 'tax.' *Om Mani Padme Hung,*" or "This is my son's demand. *Om Mani Padme Hung.*"

We, too, can use items or events in our daily life as reminders, ideally with a little purer motivation!

TYLER: You've said we should use contemplation to redirect our thoughts and then let the mind rest. Can we work with the thought process itself in letting the mind relax?

RINPOCHE: Become an astute observer of your mind. Watch the way it generates one thought after another, good and bad. Isolate a thought and observe how it catapults the mind into elation or discouragement. Then it gives way to a new thought—it's impermanent. This exercise sheds light on how the mind creates a whole reality that has no substance at all.

If you can isolate the process by which the mind solidifies the reality it projects, creating experiences and expectations, you can start to understand the illusory nature of thoughts and all they generate. Then the whole constellation of mind's habits will begin to erode. So yes, you can work this way in your contemplation. Then, when you begin to perceive the illusory nature of the thought process, let the mind rest.

~

ALTERNATING MEDITATION:
CONTEMPLATING AND RESTING

We begin by contemplating any one of Rinpoche's teachings that is particularly relevant to our current mental state or life circumstances. If and when we begin to feel tired of or overwhelmed by ideas, or no longer receptive to this line of inquiry, we drop the effort to contemplate and let the mind rest naturally—uncontrived, aware, and open—for as long as that meditative state feels truly restful.

When we notice we've become distracted or have lost awareness, we redirect our attention and open our mind to compassion in relation to the topic we've just contemplated, until the wish to end the suffering of others becomes genuine and powerful. Then we let the mind rest without effort.

Again, when our sense of spaciousness becomes crowded by thought or effort, we consider a commitment that we feel ready to make in relation to what we've contemplated. Then we let the mind rest.

As before, when the mind becomes active, we formulate a prayer in relation to the same topic. Then we let the mind rest.

We repeat this process of contemplation, compassion, commitment, and prayer—alternating each with resting the mind—as many times as we can, with each topic. We might, for example, contemplate impermanence in the context of war, generating compassion for perpetrators as well as victims, committing to resolve our own anger so that we can be a more genuine force for peace, and praying for the strength to do so, allowing the mind to rest between each step. Then we might contemplate the play of karma in our life and in the lives of others, and so forth.

If at any time in our solitary practice at home, or in our interactions with others, this sequence feels too contrived, restrictive, and effortful, we can instead change the order, or simply emphasize the steps that are most helpful in the moment. We might, for example, give rise to compassion in relation to something we've observed, or pray that the causes and conditions of someone's suffering be swiftly uprooted, and then rest the mind. As long as we alternate one or more of these methods with a state of rest, our mind will remain flexible, fresh, and deeply receptive to the impact of the meditations.

EFFORTLESS MEDITATION

Allowing the mind to rest, we don't generate, pursue, or indulge any thoughts or emotions—happy or sad, of past or future events. We don't try to find, identify, or maintain a state of rest. Rather, we simply let the mind remain spacious, open, wakeful. We neither push thoughts away, nor suppress, react to, judge, or engage them.

When a thought or emotion arises, we look directly at it: does it have a solid basis, is it illusory, dreamlike? If we are unable to discover its foundation, we rest that effort to find in the not-finding.

If and when our mind again becomes filled with a jumble of thoughts and we can't establish or continue in the state of rest, we don't waste our time judging, fighting, regretting, or rejecting what's arising. Instead, we return to the "Alternating Meditation: Contemplating and Resting" (p. 183) to refine away the extremes of conceptualization and mental dullness, until within our practice of bodhicitta we can, over time, reveal the natural, spacious awareness of our true nature.

THE NATURE OF MIND'S POISONS

When anger, desire, pride, or jealousy flood the mind, we first remind ourselves of the consequences of indulging them. Rather than succumbing to their influence, we antidote each in turn, alternating with resting the mind (p. 138).

Then we practice recognizing that they are dreamlike, that they have no solidity. And again rest the mind.

Finally, we examine them carefully. For example, when gripped by desire, we can ask ourselves, what is it? Where is it? Can we find an entity called desire with a tangible shape, size, location, and origin? If we discover that we can't find it, that's it—we've found it.

Without following the push or pull of conceptualization, we let the mind rest in recognition of the empty essence of desire's illusory display. In that openness, after repeated practice, it is possible to glimpse desire's true nature—discriminating wisdom—unlocking and freeing the appearance of desire itself. We repeat this process with each of the poisons.

12

Precious Human Birth

IMAGINE TRYING TO STAY AFLOAT on a huge ocean. You toss about, desperately attempting not to sink. Yet if a boat passes by, instead of reaching for a life preserver, a rope, or a hand to pull you up, you grab an anchor, which only drags you further down. This is our reality. Samsara is like drowning in the ocean; human existence is like resurfacing to take a breath. With spiritual methods, we can stop ourselves from going under again.

This human body is a tremendous resource. Throughout the world, we see the magnificent accomplishments that intelligence and skill make possible. Our great human potential can be harnessed not simply for material development, but also to benefit beings. Wasting this precious opportunity would be like throwing a wish-fulfilling jewel into the trash or using a big chunk of gold as a doorstop. We may not be able to accomplish all our worldly goals, but we do have the ability to overcome our suffering and that of others.

Imagine that you have labored hard at your job, year after year, and one day your boss rewards you by giving you the afternoon off. So you go on a picnic with your best friend. You lay out a blanket, unpack a delicious lunch, and open a bottle of wine. Before long, you're fighting over where to sit, who will get the drumstick, and why your friend spilled the wine. Meanwhile the sun sets, it starts to drizzle, and your picnic is over.

Human life is like such a picnic. It has taken innumerable lifetimes to finally obtain this human birth. Why waste it by fighting, criticizing, and being difficult? As much as we value our lives, so do others value theirs. As important as happiness is to us, so is it to others. If we don't use this precious opportunity to reveal our true nature, we should at least enjoy our good fortune and not spoil the experience for ourselves or others. An understanding and appreciation of the positive aspects of our lives can also help us to persevere when confronted by the waves of discouragement and despair that arise when we focus on what is wrong.

No matter how long we live, it is very difficult to purify the karma we create every day. Like someone trying to ride a bike up a steep hill, if we don't pedal vigorously, we will slide downhill fast. Without even knowing it, we cause so much harm by our very existence that we have to work diligently to resist the downhill slide. But if we apply ourselves well, we can make great gains.

Otherwise, it is as if we live in a country where we are surrounded by poisonous snakes, brigands, and murderers. A huge body of water prevents us from getting to another land beyond danger. Although someone offers us the use of a boat, we put the journey off each day until finally the owner takes his boat back.

We have this body for only a short time. If we don't use it now to get to safety, we will remain trapped in samsara with little opportunity to escape. Only the human realm offers the right combination of circumstances to do so. We experience just enough suffering that we don't easily fall prey to too much false contentment and have the incentive to undertake spiritual practice. Our moments of happiness afford us sufficient relief from suffering that we can feel compassion and engage in such practice. Although some of us are so happy that we never think about tomorrow, and some too miserable to see beyond our own pain, the human experience is the most conducive to working toward liberation from samsara.

In the lower realms, by contrast, brutality, pain, and ignorance preclude even having the concept of selflessness, much less actually considering the needs of others. Think how difficult it is to feel concern for those around us when we are sick or even slightly irritated. Imagine how much harder this would be in the lower realms. For those in the midst of such extreme suffering, there are no opportunities or resources to support outer and inner change. In the higher realms, the problem is not suffering but contentment. The gods are too drunk with pleasure to think of helping others or creating virtue, much less breaking free of samsara altogether. They never consider tomorrow, never consider that they are using up all of their positive karma only to inevitably fall into a lower existence. So rebirth in neither the lower nor higher realms is fortunate, because without feeling concern for others, we cannot awaken from the dream.

We humans have the perfect physical and mental makeup for changing the ordinary mind and revealing its true nature, enough freedom to determine the direction of our existence, and access to methods for completely transcending suffering. In this precious human life, we can use our body, speech, and mind negatively, to cause harm to ourselves and others; positively, to increase our good qualities in order to create more benefit; or ultimately, to find lasting happiness beyond the fleeting, unstable, and cyclic experiences of pleasure and pain within samsara.

Many people mistakenly believe that, having once attained a human birth, they will always be born human and that the conditions of their future lives will continually improve. They sleep comfortably at night thinking that existence is evolutionary. But this is not the case. We cannot assume that our next life will be as good as, much less better than, this one. We cannot even assume that we will be born human next time around.

Those of us who contemplate these teachings with an open mind and with the aspiration to benefit others enjoy a precious human birth. Not only are all of our mental faculties intact, but we are also receptive and connected to an unbroken lineage of the Buddha's teachings, and the conditions of our lives permit us to practice those teachings. Such a birth is as rare as a star in the noonday sky.

It was not by mere luck that we attained this birth. In previous lives, aspiring to do so, we developed a karmic connection to these truths, accumulated a vast amount of merit, and practiced moral discipline, abandoning the ten nonvirtuous actions of body, speech, and mind. If we committed any of these actions, we confessed them with sincere regret and purified them.

A precious human birth is endowed with eighteen characteristics, none of which exist in the hell, hungry ghost, animal, or god realms, for the reasons we discussed. We do not live in an eon when no buddha appeared, in a culture that embraces wrong view (for example, the idea that murder is virtuous), or where the teachings are unavailable. We as individuals are not bound by wrong view. We do not have mental or physical disabilities so severe that we cannot listen to teachings, ask questions, or contemplate. In our present eon, a buddha appeared, taught the dharma (the Buddhist teachings), and the teachings have been maintained. Though the Buddha Shakyamuni is no longer alive, others continue to apply his teachings and provide a living example of spiritual practice. We are connected to his tradition through a teacher. We have a human body with faculties intact, a tendency toward virtue and benefit, and a penetrating mind, as well as enough faith to want to explore and learn spiritual truths. We have access to these teachings and enjoy a lifestyle that is conducive to, rather than conflicts with, spiritual practice.

Many people say to me, "I know that I'm on this earth for a reason, but I'm not sure what it is." Some people think that making money and acquiring possessions are most important. Yet when we die, we won't take anything with us. No one ever has or ever will. Some people think that becoming famous, honored, and remembered once they are gone is important. But such rewards are ephemeral and may only cause jealousy. Some people think that their purpose is to write books or make beautiful music. In one way, there is virtue in bringing happiness to others through artistic endeavors. However, such pleasure is short-lived.

As much as we may try to find fulfillment in relationships, wealth, fame, or power, these are all impermanent and unreliable. The body itself is subject to sickness, old age, and death. We can find true fulfillment and freedom only by revealing the true nature of mind. Only mind's nature is reliable, infallible, and unaffected by fluctuating causes and conditions. The greatest purpose of a precious human birth is not to achieve any outer goal, but to reveal and stabilize our realization of that nature until it remains our ongoing experience. That is enlightenment—the awakened state, a state of complete freedom. With this freedom, we can ceaselessly benefit whosoever sees, hears, touches, or remembers us.

Our precious human existence is a unique vehicle for this special journey. Greater than Aladdin's lamp or a wish-fulfilling jewel, it offers the possibility of transcending all suffering and delusion, and revealing our inherent perfection. If we don't take advantage of it, we are like a poor person who returns home empty-handed from an island covered with gold, diamonds, and jewels.

If you are participating in this training, you have probably already begun dedicating your life to helping others. I deeply respect what you are doing. But it is very important that, in the process, you not become mired in mind's poisons. Please remember that rather than creating only temporary benefit, if you also use your life to attain enlightenment, your ability to benefit others will increase immeasurably.

ANGELA: I have a friend who is so unhappy that she often thinks of killing herself. She definitely doesn't think of her human life as special.

RINPOCHE: It is hard for us who live in prosperous countries to grasp how fortunate we are. If we really understood our great fortune compared with that of other humans and nonhumans, the thought of suicide would never arise.

The mind has tremendous powers of magnification. When some minor thing doesn't go our way, we see it as a big deal. Focusing on it from morning to night, we become more and more agitated and our aversion grows. If we are grazed by an arrow, that slight wound isn't so bad. But we tend to pick up the arrows of experience and stab ourselves with them over and over. How could this have happened to me? Why did he do that? Our wounds become part of our meditation: we touch them, rub salt in them, and brood over them. Such self-centeredness, combined with feelings of powerlessness, increasingly disturbs the mind. The more we dwell on our problems, the worse they seem. Viewed under a microscope, a crack in a teacup seems like the Grand Canyon. Similarly, when we obsess about our problems, they can seem so insurmountable that death appears to be the only option.

Your friend doesn't understand that if she throws her life away, it will be very, very difficult to find such a fortunate birth again. Suicide is not an escape into peaceful oblivion, but rather leads to vastly greater suffering. We don't want to be like blind sheep seeking a better pasture when we are already in the best one. Acting out of aversion to this life, attachment to death, and ignorance of the consequences of suicide, we'll find that the only doorways left open are those leading to the lower realms—the animal, hungry ghost, and hell realms. No matter how bad life is, suicide is like jumping out of a pan into the torture of a blazing fire.

Maybe you can help your friend think about it in another way. If we are sick, focusing only on our illness will soon make us feel twice as bad. Just by taking our mind off our condition, we'll feel halfway cured. Looking beyond ourselves to contemplate the suffering of others will help put our situation in perspective and allow us to appreciate our good fortune. We can break the fixation on our problems and lead the mind out of the quicksand of self-interest through compassion and prayer.

DARYL: How do I stop my feelings of despair from ruining the picnic? For example, I go for a walk in the country, but my sadness over the destruction of the environment prevents me from enjoying the beautiful surroundings.

RINPOCHE: Knowing that there are methods for reducing suffering, we don't need to despair. If we are aware of the tragic dimensions of life, we will apply those methods more diligently.

For some, to understand that human existence is a picnic means simply to enjoy it. But those who have taken these teachings to heart realize that it provides a unique opportunity to awaken. We don't know what kind of dream our mind will project when this life is over. We may not have another chance.

∾

CONTEMPLATING PRECIOUS HUMAN BIRTH

We can examine the qualities of our precious human birth both at home and in the world, alternating our contemplations with resting the mind. We think about our own life, then the lives of those we know, and finally the lives of those we have only heard or read about. Do we each enjoy most or all of the eighteen characteristics of a precious human birth?

Might the choices we are making and the way we are living lead to a precious human birth in the future?

Even if we don't believe in rebirth, we can examine whether we and others are living in such a way as to have no regrets at death. Are we fulfilling our life's purpose?

13

Impermanence

THIS RARE AND TREASURED human existence will not last forever. Our physical body is impermanent. Our parents did a little bit of this and that, and so we were conceived. We went through childhood and adolescence. Each day we grow older, and one day we will die; our body will no longer exist. Our mental capabilities are also impermanent. As we mature they increase, but later in life they decline. Our values change as well. When we were infants, our mother was all that mattered. As we got older, toys, other children, and then school captured our attention. Later, our interests shifted to romantic partners, marriage, and work. How often do we think of our mother now?

Though I am called Chagdud Tulku, I am not the same Chagdud Tulku who drank my mother's milk, caused her to spank me, or threw rocks at my neighbors. Now I am the Chagdud Tulku who teaches peace.

When we observe how change takes place in others' lives, we can begin to apply the lesson to ourselves, to realize that our bodies, too, have an expiration date. Think about all the powerful, wise, and holy people who are now just historical figures, whose lives have become no more than cherished stories. Like them, we will die. We don't know how, when, or where, but we are fooling ourselves if we assume that death lies in the distant future. Every day, we see the truth of impermanence. We can read about it in the papers or watch it on television: someone has died, an airplane has crashed, a country has been ravaged by war.

Everything in our lives—possessions, wealth, relationships—is temporary and constantly changing. Our body, speech, mind, and environment change minute by minute, second by second. In the time it takes a needle to pierce a stack of sixty flower petals cupped like spoons, not one thing in the universe stays the same. Our worst enemy could someday become our best friend, our best friend eventually our worst enemy. Husbands and wives, so in love that they cannot bear to spend an hour apart, might after a few years be repulsed by the very sight of each other. There is nothing that is not fluctuating, decaying, or transforming.

Life is unpredictable, our mental processes unstable. Our moods are susceptible to outer conditions. One morning, we may wake up feeling content; everything seems to be going beautifully. Then someone calls us with shocking news, and suddenly we're miserable. If someone pays us a compliment, we are very pleased. If somebody is insulting to us, we become furious.

Every movement we make involves change. Every sentence we utter leads to the next, the preceding one gone. Every thought or emotion gives way to another, and what came before vanishes. This happens with everything, everywhere. We simply aren't attuned to the process. We assume that something will last until, all at once, we notice it has grown old. From the moment a house is constructed, it starts deteriorating. In a hundred years or less, it will be sadly dilapidated.

Once there were no freeways; now there are thousands. Once there were very few people; now millions throng huge metropolises. Once the universe did not exist; then it came into being, and someday it will cease, along with everything in it. The seasons change, day becomes night, subatomic particles transmute and decay.

Though we devote our life to following our urges and satisfying our cravings, whatever happiness we find is fleeting. We make plans, relying on things that constantly slip through our fingers. Before we know it, they will be distant memories. How often have we been happy? How often have we been sad? Joy and sorrow come and go all the time. Neither lasts very long. Every emotion, every passion, like a drawing traced by a finger on water, is momentarily visible, then vanishes.

We need to realize that we have neither freedom not control. We can't choose how long we will live or how we will die. We don't want to get old, yet we age. We don't want to get sick, yet we become ill. We don't want to die, yet death is inevitable. It could come at any time; whether we are young, old, healthy, or ill is irrelevant.

There is nothing more traumatic than leaving our body, because there is nothing we are more attached to. We tend to take it for granted, but when impermanence overtakes us and we face death, our attachment becomes overpowering. No matter how wonderful our family, career, or possessions are, we'll take none of them with us through the doorway of death. And the day after we die, our loved ones won't even want our corpse in the house.

We have had so many bodies over innumerable lifetimes that if they were piled one on top of the other, they would resemble a great mountain. We have shed oceans of tears, committed good and bad actions beyond number, and died countless times.

Throughout all of these lives, we have suffered because of attachment. If we understand that the objects of our attachment are like mirages or bubbles, our attachment will loosen. If we know that every relationship is fragile and likely to change, we will realize there is no time for conflict. If we truly comprehend that we cannot count on even one more day, at least we won't destroy our own and others' chances to enjoy this life while we have it.

Knowing that each moment might be our last puts things into perspective. We won't think about the imperfections of our existence when death is imminent. When our loved ones die, it will be too late to cry or feel regret over things undone or unsaid. Now is the time to cherish them, not after they are gone.

Reflecting on impermanence changes our habit of clinging to things as stable and immutable. For example, if as we put the key in the ignition of our expensive new car, we remind ourselves that it is just a box of rust waiting to happen, our attachment to it will diminish. We may meet a wonderful person and hope that she is the one for us. This is when we need to recall that everything is impermanent.

Some people think that the idea of impermanence is depressing, but actually it's the truth of our experience. Just as fire is hot and water wet, impermanence is just the way things are; it's neither good nor bad. Accepting it cures us of our wishful thinking that we can stave off the inexorable process of change and gives us a greater capacity for acceptance and joy. No matter how difficult or painful our circumstances may be, as long as we are on this side of death, they aren't that bad. Instead of feeling discouraged by impermanence, we can rejoice, thinking, "I'm alive. I'm with my friends and family. I have a wonderful opportunity to do spiritual practice, to benefit others."

Contemplating impermanence has been a tremendous support in my own life. When I was three years old, I was recognized as the *tulku*—or reincarnation—of the previous Chagdud Tulku, and at four began training intensively with a tutor. Every day and evening, without any time off, I sat with him and studied. I often watched children romping outside, thinking how fortunate they were to be playing together. I wanted to join them in their games, and I missed my mother. During this period, I started receiving teachings on impermanence. I didn't have much choice—if I didn't listen, I was punished. Luckily, I wasn't one to do things in a superficial way, so I really probed their meaning.

My tutor told me that the more I reflected on impermanence, the more I would be able to use my precious human existence to help others. Especially as a tulku, I needed to accomplish something of benefit in this lifetime. Despite my youth, sick people came to me, asking that I pray for them. Whenever someone died, the body was brought to me to be blessed before being buried or cremated. So I knew everyone who was sick and everyone who died. I saw very clearly that life is fragile.

At the age of nine, I began to receive formal meditation instruction. I learned that for something to be absolutely true, it has to be permanent, singular, and unaffected by anything else. I looked at life carefully and began to see that nothing meets these criteria.

When I was eleven, my mother put me in my first three-year retreat. Day in and day out without a break, I studied and meditated in a monastery with people of all ages. My mother told me to practice no matter what happened, because then I would be able to benefit others. She spoke of impermanence so often that some people began to think she might not live much longer. A few months later, she died in childbirth.

At first I was in shock. There was no way at that age that I could comprehend my mother's death. When I heard the news, my first thought was "This is the meaning of impermanence." I had lost my mother and realized that I, too, would die, and so would everyone else. The assumption that I could count on anything in life was shattered. I didn't get angry at the world for being impermanent. I simply came to the realization that nothing is reliable.

At eleven, I had become the decision maker for my baby brother, sister, and other family members. My mother had left quite a bit behind—hundreds of yaks and dozens of horses. She had been building an enormous prayer wheel, and her last wish was that it be completed. So I used all of her wealth for this purpose. Now not only was my mother gone, but so were most of our possessions. Only six yaks and two horses remained. This succession of changes took place so quickly, it was dreamlike.

When I turned twelve, my little brother, to whom I was very attached, drowned. I loved my mother and brother tremendously, but because of my training in impermanence, their deaths didn't overwhelm me.

The more I contemplated, the more everything seemed illusory. I understood how easy it is to lose this precious human life. Because I knew it wouldn't last long, I took joy in each new day. I rejoiced each morning—how wonderful that I hadn't died in my sleep!

When I was thirteen, my tutor suddenly left because of a family emergency, and I never saw him again. He had been my daily companion since I was five. We had eaten, studied, and meditated together. We had even slept in the same room. Our minds were intimately connected. He had done everything a mother would do, and his kindness rivaled that of my mother.

At one time, twenty-two people in my family lived and ate together in a giant tent. All but three or four of them died during the Communist Chinese occupation of Tibet. Some died in prison, some were killed, but most died of starvation. In 1959 I escaped from Tibet, leaving everything familiar to me—my family, my monastery, my homeland.

Many of those who fled the country were strongly attached to their wealth and tried to take whatever they could on their backs or on pack animals. Because they traveled slowly and were highly visible, the Chinese often caught them, took their possessions, and killed them or threw them in jail. On the other hand, the group I traveled with left everything behind and ran; we didn't even take a change of clothes. The others thought we were crazy, but we made it to India.

Death was a constant and immediate presence in the refugee camps there. I cannot say that I didn't suffer, but because I had reflected deeply on impermanence, it was easier to bear the death, loss, and tragedy.

Now everything I do is like play. I'm not apathetic or uninvolved, but rather like an old man playing with his grandchildren. I teach, share, and try to help as much as I can without believing any of it to be permanent.

I have fully learned that if we live each day as if it were our last, we will make choices that we won't regret at the time of death. Instead of getting completely caught up in our lives, in our hopes and fears, likes and dislikes, thinking we'll practice later, we will understand that there is no time to procrastinate. Who can say that death will wait? We need to unflinchingly confront the fact that we are in a race with death. We have to act quickly, doing all we can to reduce our mental poisons and work toward realizing that which is beyond permanence and impermanence—the true nature of mind.

The great Tibetan yogi Milarepa used to meditate, naked, on a mountainside under extremely harsh conditions. His sister had given him some cloth to make robes, but when she came to see him, she saw that the cloth was unused.

"You're crazy!" she said. "With very little effort, you could have made some robes to protect yourself from the cold, wind, and snow."

However, Milarepa thought that she was the crazy one because, in itself, sewing the cloth wouldn't have brought him one step closer to enlightenment. In the time it would have taken him to make robes, he had come to the understanding in meditation that no matter how good or bad things are, they come and go. He saw no need for robes; his realization gave him all the protection he needed. By the power of his practice, he experienced warmth and bliss while sitting naked on the snow, whereas others suffer while sitting in warm clothes on soft cushions.

TERESA: Though I've had some understanding of impermanence for a while, I seem even more attached to things—to my terrific husband and my beautiful home. I've traded some involvements for others, but on the whole it feels as though my attachment has increased.

RINPOCHE: There is nothing wrong with having a nice home and a kind husband. To cut your attachment, you don't have to leave your husband or burn your house down. But you do need to abandon your assumption that things will continue as they are, as if they were solid and long lasting. A child chasing a rainbow, thinking it something substantial, is sure she can catch it. But no matter how much she tries, she never will.

Cutting attachment requires knowing that everything—your husband, the house, *everything*—is impermanent. Whatever you experience, never forget that it will change. That's the way of the world. This understanding will enable you to appreciate what you have, to enjoy it while it lasts. When you lose something, you won't be taken by surprise, because you won't have assumed it could never be lost. People leave, houses deteriorate, and everyone dies. As long as you understand impermanence, these things won't break you.

ANGELA: Why would we bother with anything at all if everything is impermanent?

RINPOCHE: The point is that we need to recognize the impermanence of the things in our life, not to throw everything out the window. As long as we still have desire, that strategy will backfire. Before long, regret will set in and we'll feel the need to replace everything we've thrown out because our desires still haven't been fulfilled.

We have to realize that there is nothing much about our shiny new car we can hold on to, that we aren't much more than a caretaker paying for insurance. With anything new, we should remind ourselves from the start that someday we'll lose it, if only at death. Then, when we do, we won't be taken by surprise or be so disturbed.

Knowing that nothing lasts lends equilibrium to our lives. We realize that whatever happens, good or bad, is impermanent—eventually the pendulum will swing the other way. We know that the more attached we are to something, the more miserable we'll be when it's gone. We don't reject happiness just because we know that it's impermanent; rather, we become less attached to the conditions that have produced it. If we aren't as upset when things change, we can tell that our contemplation of impermanence is effective.

SARAH: My parents fought incessantly throughout my childhood and still do. I've tried to help in many ways, but nothing works. I feel hopeless about their lives ever changing. It seems that their suffering is the one exception to impermanence.

RINPOCHE: Your parents' fighting and the suffering it causes are as impermanent as anything else. Even if they fought eight hours a day, there may have been moments when they were happy together. Maybe when they made love, they gave each other joy.

Try not to be disheartened by the fact that you haven't been able to change their situation. If it were possible to end others' suffering, the buddhas and bodhisattvas would already have done so, because their aspiration to help others is boundless, beyond our ability to imagine. But all beings, like your parents, are subject to the laws of karma.

To help your parents, you can pray, meditate, and dedicate merit. This may not seem very effective, but don't be discouraged. In the same way that seeds beneath the ground aren't visible, the blessings of prayer and meditation may not be immediately apparent. But just as seeds eventually germinate, your efforts will one day come to fruition.

DARYL: I'm not convinced that contemplating impermanence will make me more compassionate.

RINPOCHE: When we truly realize that everything is impermanent, we naturally feel compassion for others because we see that people's belief in the solidity of their experience—their clinging to it as something stable and reliable—causes them to suffer. Awareness of impermanence and the compassion it arouses become the foundation of our life and spiritual practice.

~

CONTEMPLATING IMPERMANENCE

We begin our contemplation of impermanence by examining every aspect of our experience—the universe, the earth, our neighborhood, our relationships, our body, speech, and mind, our interests and values, even our self-identity—to see if we can find anything that does not change. We contemplate each, then let the mind rest, continuing with the "Alternating Meditation: Contemplating and Resting" (p. 183) during our formal practice sessions or when the circumstances of our informal practice allow.

By truly assimilating the meaning of impermanence through contemplation and meditation, over time we will grasp less at things that will certainly fail us, and establish the basis for the state of peace we so desperately seek.

THE RATE OF CHANGE

In this meditation, instead of using the conceptual mind to think about impermanence, we simply pay attention and open, through all our senses, to the rate and process of change around us. If we find ourselves lost in thoughts or emotions related to the past or future, we remind ourselves that those thoughts themselves are an example of impermanence. We were aware of changes taking place within and around us, then we lost that awareness, and now we'll reestablish it by bringing ourselves back to the present moment. We then continue to observe directly that whatever happens doesn't last very long—each and every moment is fleeting, illusory, and can't be grasped. We repeat this exercise as often as possible and in different settings throughout the day.

FINDING THE PRESENT MOMENT

Considering that the past has come and gone, and the future has not yet arisen, we try to find the present moment. Can we capture it? If we think we've found it, we need to look more deeply. Does it have a beginning, middle, and end? Is there any instant that isn't in the process of change?

In our search for the present moment, if we feel confused or lost, we let go of the effort to find it and let the mind rest. Or if we think we've found it, we rest there.

14

Karma

WHEN I WAS TWENTY-FIVE or so, I undertook a retreat at a remote site on a holy mountain in central Tibet. The lama overseeing my retreat advised me not to take any money along because people in the area had been known to rob and kill practitioners. He said that he knew of a sponsor who would send me all the food I might need.

So off I went to retreat with just a small bag of *tsampa* (roasted barley flour), which I planned to eat with a little butter and tea, as is the Tibetan custom. As time passed, I ate the tsampa without thinking much about it until it was half gone. I still hadn't received anything from my sponsor, but there was nothing I could do at that point. I had made a commitment not to leave retreat for any reason whatsoever.

So I cut down my ration of tsampa to one small cup a day. When it ran out, I had no food for many days. All my dreams and visions indicated that my practice was good and my needs would be met. There were heaps of food in my dreams, and I sometimes found a few potatoes or small amounts of tsampa outside my door in the morning, but they weren't enough. I became very weak and had to be careful when I stood up so as not to pass out.

One day a lama who was in retreat nearby came to visit. He wanted to meet me because we were both from eastern Tibet. When he discovered that I had no food, he went off and returned with some soup. Each day thereafter, I had a lunch guest who furnished the meal. Eventually my sponsor remembered me. He apologized profusely and sent regular supplies for the rest of my retreat.

This is the power of karma. I had a generous sponsor who was willing to feed me well but forgot. I could have provided for myself with my own money, but hadn't brought any with me. If I had known before I'd made the commitment not to leave my retreat that I would be without food, I could have gone begging. Everything seemed to go wrong in a way that no one could have foreseen, because what happened was simply the playing out of karma. I could have blamed my sponsor, but it wasn't really his fault.

When I escaped from Tibet with a group of five, including my elderly teacher and his brother, we moved from place to place in the forest, dodging the Communist Chinese soldiers. We waited until winter to cross the border into India because we knew the Indian heat would kill us. We had lost everything but five hundred Chinese silver coins. With some of these we bought corn, which we used to make soup mixed with greens that we gathered in the woods.

My teacher and I were having dreams about loss. It was difficult for us to take them seriously because we'd already lost almost everything. But they occurred night after night, so we knew that something might happen. We also had dreams indicating that we should change locations, so we left our heavy packs in a nearby town and moved on. I had always carried the silver

coins on my body, but this time decided to leave all but fifty in my pack so that I could move quickly. I intended to retrieve them later. The next morning, before dawn, I heard gunshots coming from the town where we had left our packs. The Chinese had taken the town.

I am telling you these stories so that you won't get discouraged when things go badly, but instead will persevere. Even if we have the wisdom to see what is coming, we cannot escape our karma. The only thing to do is to purify it before it ripens.

Many successful people think the reason they have done so well in life is that they are smart and skilled in business. But many smart, skillful people are also poor, so something more than intelligence and talent is required for success. Some people work hard to make money and eventually prosper but, when they invest their earnings, lose everything. Or they may be robbed, even killed, for their wealth. Others succeed without much effort at all—things just go well for them.

Some people are preoccupied with their health. They take all the right vitamins, exercise regularly, and eat well, yet are sick most of the time. Others never exercise, and consume as much salt and sugar as they want, yet remain in perfect health.

This is all because of karma.

Sometimes a minor illness can result in death. A friend of mine, though he felt perfectly healthy, was told by a doctor that a small spot on his lung had to be removed. The doctor assured him that he would be hospitalized for no more than two or three days. While my friend was in the hospital, complications set in and he died.

I once knew a woman who had endured thirteen miscarriages. When she became pregnant a fourteenth time, her doctor, believing her health to be at risk, gave her a drug to terminate the pregnancy. She put the pills in her medicine cabinet. The next day she took them, but they didn't work, and nine months later she gave birth to a healthy baby. It turned out that she had mixed up the bottles in her medicine cabinet and taken the wrong drug. The first thirteen babies hadn't had the karma to come into this world. But nothing could stop the fourteenth from being born, because that was the child's karma.

So what is karma, this unbending principle that accounts for everything that happens, good or bad? Imagine a seagull casting a shadow while he stands on a rock. When he flies away, he thinks he has no shadow, but as soon as he lands, there it is again. The effects of our actions follow us like shadows, whether we realize it or not.

A single seed will produce a whole tree with many branches, flowers, and fruit, and each fruit will contain even more seeds. The smallest seed of anger will produce great suffering for ourselves and others. By the same token, even a small act of generosity or compassion will produce great happiness. We usually don't know what will come from the seeds we sow. They lie dormant in the mind for a long time, and when they finally begin to sprout, we have forgotten having planted them at all. Eventually, though, they will bear fruit.

Think of it this way: Sometime in the past, we wrote a book, recording every one of our thoughts—happy and unhappy, angry and pleasant—the amazing, swirling contents of our mind. After we finished, we hid the book and forgot about it.

Forty years later, we find it in the attic and start to read. We can't remember having written these things. We become totally absorbed, as if by the writing of a stranger. When we read something sad, we cry. When we read something funny, we laugh.

In the same way, we experience now what we have written karmically with our past thoughts, words, and actions. Just as we are both the writer and reader of our book, we create our karma and experience its fruits. Having forgotten the karmic tale we wrote, we may feel victimized, wishing to escape from our drama. But only by purifying our karma can we change the story line.

Almost every religion teaches this same principle: if we are good, our future experience will be positive; if we are harmful, it will be negative. In the Buddhist tradition, there are a few more stops on the journey. According to the nature of our actions, we cycle through lifetimes of happiness, unhappiness, or a mixture of both. This goes on and on unless we transform the mind and awaken to enlightenment.

But no matter what your spiritual path may be, if you refrain from harming and try to help others, your future experience and that of those around you will improve. Not harming others is like not drinking poison. Helping others is like taking medicine.

THE INTRICACIES OF KARMA

Buddhism teaches that the full ripening of an act involves four steps. In the case of killing, the first step involves identifying the object—the being we want to kill, like an insect eating the flowers in our garden. The second step consists of formulating the intention to kill: "You are going to die, aphids, not my flowers!" The third is the act of murder itself. The fourth is the consequence, the death of the victim.

The process works the same way if the action is virtuous. First, we identify the person we wish to benefit and generate the intention to do so. Then we do something on his behalf, and he receives the benefit.

If you identify an enemy, have the intention to kill him, do everything you can to succeed but fail, three of the four steps are involved. Accidentally stepping on an insect doesn't entail the first two steps. But squashing it involves the third, and its death, the fourth. The repercussions in such a case are much less severe than when something involves all four steps.

Traditionally, it is said that any act that includes these four steps produces a "fully ripened result"—for example, rebirth in a hell realm in the case of murder motivated by anger or desire. After this result come "experiences similar to the cause," in which, in our example, the murderer spends five hundred lifetimes as a human with a very short life span, being repeatedly killed in ways similar to the way he had killed. Then follows the experience of "actions similar to the cause," in which the momentum of the murderer's karma manifests as a behavioral pattern similar to those in his previous lives. As a young child, he might abuse other children or torture animals. Finally, there is the "conditioning result," rebirth in an environment that reflects the mental poison that motivated the initial harmful action, such as a place with extremely harsh conditions.

Negative karma is created by the three nonvirtues of body, the four nonvirtues of speech, and the three nonvirtues of mind. The physical nonvirtues include killing, stealing, and sexual misconduct. We can kill someone out of anger, desire, or simply a lack of consideration for life—for example, by sweeping an insect away as we clean the floor. The karmic consequences are more severe and long lasting if we act out of desire, and more serious still if we are motivated by anger.

Stealing means taking anything not given to us. It also includes taking something against someone's will or behind someone's back, overpricing an item, tricking someone into believing that an item is worth more than it is (or that we paid more for it than we did), exaggerating the quantity or quality of something, or accepting payment for services based on misrepresentation of our qualifications.

Sexual misconduct includes breaking commitments, such as a monk's or nun's vow of celibacy or a layperson's commitment to his partner. Sexual activity that harms another—for example, with someone who is sick or underage—is also misconduct, as is interfering with someone else's relationship.

The nonvirtues of speech begin with lying or leading someone to believe something that isn't true. Claiming to be something we are not when people rely on us—for example, claiming to be a great doctor and lying about our credentials—is especially serious.

Slander includes causing divisions among friends. This is particularly nonvirtuous among spiritual practitioners, bound by their sacred commitments to respect and honor each other.

Harsh speech includes yelling and cursing, as well as pointing out someone's faults in a way that hurts her feelings or exposes her shortcomings. Knives, swords, stones, and guns can hurt only the body, but harmful speech acts like a razor blade on the mind.

Gossip refers to any useless speech. It includes spreading rumors, as well as mindless babbling that distracts others' attention and wastes not only the gossip's time, but his listeners' as well. Useless speech is particularly nonvirtuous if it keeps someone from spiritual practice or distracts her from recognition of her true nature.

The three nonvirtues of mind are covetousness, wishing that someone else's good fortune were our own; harmful thought, which includes rejoicing in the misfortune of others or wishing them harm; and wrong view, such as thinking that virtue is nonvirtuous or vice versa.

Each of the ten nonvirtues has a corresponding virtue. Instead of taking life, we can save it. Whether we ransom beings and let them go free or care for them, saving life helps to balance the nonvirtue of taking life. Every year, I undertake the practice of saving lives. I go to the ocean, to the bait stores on the dock. I buy live bait and then release it into the ocean, offering prayers and dedicating the virtue to the long life of all beings, wherever they exist in samsara.

Instead of stealing, we can give. We can uphold our commitments concerning sexual conduct. We can use our speech in a virtuous, gentle, and honest way to create harmony and unity; we can also chant mantra and read spiritual texts. The words of sacred texts have a great impact on those who hear them— human and nonhuman alike—so there is enormous benefit in reciting them aloud.

A great scholar living in India used to recite a particular scripture over and over again. One day, halfway through the recitation, a baby bird flew out of a nest near his open window and was killed by a hawk. The bird took rebirth as the son of a king in another country, and at a very young age started reciting the first half of the same scripture. He asked, "Where is my lama? He can teach me the other half."

Inquiries were made, and an Indian scholar renowned for reciting this scripture was located. The prince traveled to India and immediately recognized the scholar. "My lama!" he exclaimed. "I am so happy to see you."

By virtue of having heard just half of the scripture, the bird had been reborn as a human who remembered his previous life and could thus find his teacher and study with him. Eventually, he became a great scholar himself.

Instead of coveting what others have, we can rejoice in their happiness and virtue. We can think kind and loving thoughts, and develop a clear understanding of and appreciation for spiritual truths.

All such virtuous actions of body, speech, and mind will antidote our nonvirtuous actions and unfailingly produce happiness in the future.

We need to consider carefully what is beneficial and how we can be of greatest service. We share the world with other human beings, so we must learn to avoid situations that we know will have a negative impact. We establish the intention not to harm others, and we constantly examine ourselves, making adjustments when necessary. If we see that something will not benefit either temporarily or ultimately, we make a commitment not to do it.

SARAH: So I'm the one to blame for my problems? Doesn't someone who harms me have some responsibility?

RINPOCHE: When we are in the midst of a problem, what we experience is due to our karma. Without the karmic cause, no outer condition could have produced these circumstances. Our efforts to understand and deal with the pain tempt us to blame others. But pointing the finger at someone else, or reacting with anger or resentment, only perpetuates the problem and creates more nonvirtue. The principle of karma forces us to take responsibility for our own and others' suffering. We misunderstand it if we use it to justify blame.

On the other hand, a person who harms us bears responsibility for the resulting karma even if he doesn't realize it. Karma is like a dance—one person moves forward, the other moves back, the dancers interdependent, like everything in the dream of existence. If you offer someone tea, eventually it will come back to you. Any cup of tea offered to you is yours by virtue of your previous generosity.

HELEN: A friend of mine was hit by a drunk driver. How could anyone say that this was her fault? Wouldn't that be cold and uncompassionate?

RINPOCHE: The fault lies with karma. But it is important to clearly understand what I am going to say so that you don't mistakenly adopt a fatalistic approach. All of our circumstances arise from karmic seeds that we have planted in the past, but we still have the ability to determine our future experience. In some previous life, your friend harmed someone, and the resulting karma led to her present situation. She is not aware of what she did, but can't escape the consequences.

Karma is unyielding and brutal, but if we understand how it works, we can change its course. This is because in reacting to our present karma as it ripens, we make more karma, which will affect our future. That karma is either positive or negative, depending on how we choose to respond. The only way to break the perpetual cycle of action and reaction is to make different choices.

SARAH: How can you explain karma to children who have been beaten or sexually abused?

RINPOCHE: Speaking to them about karma won't help, because it won't mean anything to them. Instead, urge them to be positive and not let the abuser's actions fill them with hatred as well. The best approach is to help them realize that the experience is over. Your love and compassion are the best medicine.

ORLIN: In counseling her patients, a family therapist would say that all family members should look at themselves and take responsibility for their own behavior and feelings. Is this what you would recommend?

RINPOCHE: This is an important point. Many people blame their parents for their problems. But our parents aren't really to blame. When we were conceived, they didn't pull us out of the intermediate state so they could torture us. Our karma brought us to them. Out of billions of people, two became our parents, and not by accident.

Some people think that they consciously chose their parents, but that isn't true either. We didn't choose our parents; they didn't choose us. We didn't want to suffer, nor did they want to make us suffer. We are connected to one another by karma. If our parents have shortcomings or our relationship is difficult, it is ultimately not their fault. It is the result of our karma. We must look beyond the immediate moment to see our relationships from a broader perspective.

TYLER: How do we make so much karma?

RINPOCHE: If the mind perceives an object and remains in a state of relaxation, we won't make karma. But usually the mind becomes involved with the outer stimulus, believing it to be inherently real. We respond to it with attachment or aversion, reacting with body, speech, or mind. We do this every moment of our existence, lifetime after lifetime.

In each instant, we have the potential either to awaken or to become lost in the movement of ordinary mind. We always have that choice. Ultimately, the mind never moves from its true nature. But its apparent motion leads us to identify with the ordinary mind, without awareness of its nature.

That nature is not a void, like a blackboard that has been erased. With its rich potential for expression, it is the basis of all phenomena—everything arises from it. When we stabilize the realization that the unlimited expression of mind is never separate from its nature, we stop creating karma.

VINCENT: Do the karmic seeds we plant bear fruit in one lifetime or several lifetimes later?

RINPOCHE: Generally, karma doesn't ripen in just one, but over many lifetimes, though sometimes spiritual practice accelerates the process.

There was a great lama from my region in Tibet who endured ill health for more than twenty years. His meditative realization was such that he could remember a previous lifetime in which he had killed a musk deer for the glands used in producing incense. He knew that his poor health in this life was the consequence of that act.

For karma to ripen, there must be both cause and conditions. The conditions determine whether the ripening takes place in one lifetime or another. Any seed we have planted will lie dormant until the circumstances are right. The karma we've accumulated over lifetimes is like a mountain of seeds waiting for the right conditions to grow.

Sometimes one's karma can indeed ripen within a single lifetime. When I was about eight years old, I killed a small fish, though because of my training, I knew better than to do so. Years later, during my second three-year retreat, I dreamt of an ocean—something I'd never seen—and a voice that said, "This is where you will be reborn." I realized that as a result of having killed the fish, I would be reborn as one. I prayed, "May I be a small fish, so that I don't create negative karma as a predator."

When I woke up the next morning, it was still dark, but everywhere I turned I saw the fish. I decided to recite *Om Mani Padme Hung*—the mantra of Avalokiteshvara, the bodhisattva of compassion—a hundred thousand times each day, in between meditation sessions. I dedicated the virtue of this practice to the fish I'd killed and made the aspiration that, no matter where it had been reborn, it might be released from suffering. After about five or six days, the visions dissolved, but I continued saying the mantra until I had completed a million recitations.

ALEXANDRA: How can we suffer in hell from actions that we didn't know were wrong?

RINPOCHE: You don't have to know what you've done to experience its effects. You may sow seeds without your ordinary mind knowing what they will produce. Ignorance is so pervasive that we don't even register how many mistakes we make, but as we purify our obscurations, we become more aware.

ALEXANDRA: Before we come back to the human realm, do we receive instructions so that we won't repeat our negative actions?

RINPOCHE: Beings in the hell realms know why they are there. They know that it's not a mistake. My mother was a *delog,* someone who dies and then returns to report what death and the other realms are like. She told many stories of people in the hell and hungry ghost realms who knew why they were suffering. They gave her messages—including confessions or the locations of stolen goods they'd hidden—to take to living relatives, imploring them to sponsor ceremonies on their behalf.

We leave these realms with the intention to never create such nonvirtue again. But we forget, and our residual karma comes to fruition. It is hard to reverse our tendencies and temperament without spiritual methods.

TERESA: What is the relationship between one's obstacles and one's karma?

RINPOCHE: Obstacles affect us only if our karma makes us susceptible. For example, in a place like Los Angeles, with several million inhabitants, pollution doesn't have the same impact on everyone. Some people become very ill, while others are hardly affected. Our ability to overcome an obstacle depends on our karma. Sometimes we can easily change the outer conditions; if not, we need to purify the karma that led to the obstacle.

~

EXPLORING KARMA

We begin by examining some aspect of the teachings about karma—for example, the four steps involved in the full ripening of a karmic act. Through the course of our day, how often did we identify someone we wanted to help or harm, and then cultivate the intention to do so? Did we act on that intention, and did the action produce its intended result? Then, keeping in mind this examination of our daily choices of body, speech, and mind, and their intended or unintended consequences, we practice the "Alternating Meditation: Contemplating and Resting" (p. 183).

Alternating with resting the mind, we review our day by generating compassion toward those we've harmed as well as those who have, perhaps unknowingly, harmed others through their actions. We give rise to a commitment to do something differently and then pray, alternating each aspect of our meditation with resting the mind.

Next we could consider how a shift in our motivation during those same events might have produced a different result. Might this shift have produced virtue instead of nonvirtue? What if these same events had been characterized by an increase of loving kindness instead of resentment or anger? How might that have produced different outcomes?

We continue to alternate our examination of each aspect of the teachings on karma with compassion, commitment, prayer, and resting the mind, so that our understanding and acceptance of its impact on our lives increasingly informs all our actions of body, speech, and mind, producing greater benefit for ourselves and others.

KARMA AND THE SPACIOUS MIND

Repeating the meditation "How Suffering Begins" (p. 160), we observe the sequence of events that leads the mind from a state of rest to perception, judgment, the mental poisons, and finally the creation of karma. How is our current experience shaped by our habitual responses to appearances? How might our future experience change if, instead of indulging our familiar patterns of thought and emotion, we antidoted and transformed them, and acted only out of pure motivation?

We then let the mind rest.

Then we explore how our lives might change if, instead of repeating these same patterns of attachment, aversion, and reactivity, we simply let our mind remain spacious and open in every moment of our daily life, allowing our negative emotions to dissolve instead of reinforcing and perpetuating them. Then, again, we rest the mind.

15

Working with Karma in Daily Life

VINCENT: Sometimes, even though I try to do the right thing, everything goes wrong. Is this because of my karma?

RINPOCHE: For the most part, yes. Once, there was a great practitioner who lived and meditated in a forest. One day, he decided to dye his robes in a big pot on a fire and left them boiling while he went to collect more firewood. Meanwhile, a farmer who had lost a calf happened by. He peeked into the steaming pot and thought he saw his calf boiling away.

Furious, the farmer went to the king and said, "There is a man in the forest claiming to be a yogi, but he stole my calf and is cooking it. I want you to do something!"

So the king had the meditator arrested and jailed. Seven days later, the farmer found the calf. He hurried to the king to apologize and requested that the yogi be released. The king agreed to do so, but forgot. After seven months of searching, one of the yogi's students finally found him in jail. He went to the king and asked him to free his teacher. Horrified, the king himself went to the yogi and apologized, saying, "I knew seven months ago that you were innocent but forgot to release you. I am very sorry you were confined for so long."

The yogi replied, "It wasn't your fault. Many lifetimes ago, I stole a calf. As I was running from its owner, I saw a yogi sitting by the road. I threw the calf in his direction so it would look like he had stolen it. The yogi went to jail for seven days. For many eons, I purified this karma in the hell realms; now that I've found a human birth again, I have further purified it by spending seven months in jail. Because of my karma, the farmer mistook my clothes for his calf, and you forgot to release me."

We have enormous amounts of karma to purify. It will ripen despite our good heart and pure intention. Some people think that perfect health is a sign that someone is doing everything right and that the Buddhist path is somehow lacking because some practitioners become ill. When great meditators get sick, it isn't because they have done something terribly wrong in this life. Rather, their illness is exhausting karma created in past lifetimes. One yogi sang, "If I am sick, I rejoice, because my nonvirtue is being purified. If I am well, I rejoice, because I can use my body, speech, and mind to create virtue."

Be consistent and persevering. Don't become discouraged, but recognize that the real reason for your difficulties is that your negative karma is being purified.

SARAH: In trying to help a patient at work, if my intention is pure but I inadvertently say something that upsets him, will I make negative karma?

RINPOCHE: No. If your motivation is selfless, even if your efforts are not effective or end up backfiring, you won't produce negative karma. However, you have to be honest—make sure you're not acting out of attachment or aversion, hope or fear.

For example, in the case of mercy killing, you might think that your motivation is compassion, when in fact you are motivated by aversion to suffering or attachment to ending that suffering.

ANGELA: It's pretty hard for me to imagine that killing a cockroach has serious consequences.

RINPOCHE: No being wants to suffer, not even an insect. Yet we seldom consider this. If termites damage our home, we don't hesitate to kill them, thinking that eliminating such small creatures is inconsequential. When we do so out of anger or aversion, we ensure future suffering for ourselves far surpassing that of the insects we've killed.

Sometimes, out of ignorance, we simply can't avoid killing insects or destroying their homes as we walk, breathe, or drive. But we should strive not to harm anyone, no matter how small, and take every precaution to reduce the impact we have. The karmic outcome is determined not by the size of the being we kill, but by what is in our minds at the time.

ALEXANDRA: I became a vegetarian to save animals' lives, but my doctors have advised me to start eating meat again. It seems wrong for me to eat meat for what appears to be a minor health problem.

RINPOCHE: Your motivation for being a vegetarian is compassion. You don't want anything to be killed, and that is virtuous. Yet many people feel healthier when they eat meat. We create karma no matter what we eat. It's a hopeless situation, because if we don't eat we die.

Since we have to eat, how can we minimize the harm involved? The Buddha's solution was to eat only one meal a day. To Buddhists, every life is of equal value. Most Tibetans don't eat fish because usually several have to be consumed to satisfy a single person's hunger. Highlanders prefer to eat yak because twenty people can live on the meat of a single animal for twenty days. They often think of lowlanders as nonvirtuous because they kill so many beings when they plow the land—beings living in the ground, by exposing them to the elements and birds; beings living above the ground, by burying or squashing them; and even more beings during the cultivation and watering of crops. Lowlanders, on the other hand, criticize highlanders for cutting the throats of animals and watching them bleed to death.

None of these people want to create nonvirtue, but they can't avoid it. The important thing is motivation. It is highly commendable to refrain from eating meat to spare a being from suffering and death. If your intention is never to eat grains or vegetables for the same reason, that is also very good. But either way, you are in a quandary because your life depends on food.

All beings exist interdependently. Consuming the flesh of an animal, or vegetables and grains cultivated and harvested at the expense of many insects' lives, establishes a connection with those beings. To transform that negative connection into one of virtue, we acknowledge that beings have died so that we can eat. Before a meal, we offer our food—visualizing that it multiplies to fill all of space—to the object of our faith. We dedicate the merit of our offering to everyone connected to us, including the turkey in our sandwich or the insect that died while the rice was harvested. We pray that they and all beings will have fortunate rebirths, ideally as humans who discover an authentic spiritual path and the means to gain temporary and ultimate happiness. At the end of every day or at the close of a meditation session, we also dedicate our virtue. In this way, we help the beings who have died so that we may eat, live in houses, and wear clothes.

For Tibetans who are nomadic, the vow not to harm others is very difficult to keep because most of them depend on meat for their sustenance. Some families maintain the vow all year, but break it on the day they have to slaughter their animals. Only one person in the family does the butchering so that not everyone is tainted by that act.

Some Tibetans make a commitment not to kill or eat meat during certain months or on auspicious days, such as the full moon, the new moon, the eighth, tenth, twenty-first, or twenty-third day of the lunar calendar. Upholding such a vow for even one day a year is better than having no vow, intention, or aspiration.

During the Buddha's time, there lived a practitioner who, because of the power of his meditation, could travel from realm to realm. He once came upon a man who by day burned in a hot iron box while vicious dogs tore at his flesh. By night, he sat on a throne in a jeweled palace while four goddesses served him with adoration. At the break of dawn, he was thrust back into the burning box.

The practitioner asked the man what had led to such an existence. He replied that in a former life in India, he had been born into a family of butchers. One day, a disciple of the Buddha explained to him the consequences of killing. The man was convinced by what he said but, being of the butcher caste, had no other way to support his family. So he vowed that, from then on, he wouldn't kill anything as soon as night fell, even at the cost of his life. The virtue of having upheld that commitment now gave him nightly respite from his hellish suffering.

One of my students lives in a place where it is culturally unacceptable *not* to hunt. I told him to hunt only for the sake of subsistence, and not on days considered auspicious in the Buddhist tradition. When we buy meat, although an animal has died, we have not identified the being to be killed or acted with the intention to kill it. Our enjoyment of the meat is still nonvirtuous, but far less so than if we'd slaughtered the animal ourselves.

The first step on the bodhisattva path is to make the commitment not to harm others, to whatever degree that is possible. It's wonderful if you can fully uphold this commitment. Otherwise, assess what you can do. The butcher was better off vowing not to kill at night than making no vow at all. You can always do something to reduce your negative impact and to be more helpful. Whether you decide to eat meat or remain a vegetarian, don't become self-righteous. Without condemning anyone else's lifestyle, do the best you can, remembering to offer your food and dedicate the merit to those who died so that you might live.

BEN: Given the nonvirtue of killing and even of farming, would it be better if we simply ate berries and other kinds of fruit that grow wild?

RINPOCHE: If you had pure motivation and pure heart, you could reduce your nonvirtue by taking care not to step on beings in the woods and by eating berries. The Buddha himself ate only one meal a day, and only when someone offered it to him. The great yogi Milarepa wandered for many years without begging and survived on nettles. It wasn't that he couldn't get a job; he simply felt that this was the best way to keep from making negative karma. Milarepa's good heart and pure intentions made his asceticism virtuous and beneficial.

On the other hand, a healthy body supports your practice, which in turn supports others. So if you have pure motivation, caring for your body will not result in bad karma.

IMANI: I can see how karma works with individuals, but what's the karmic situation when it comes to large groups of people, as in the case of Tibet and China?

RINPOCHE: Space is filled with beings living in the six realms of experience. Those in each realm have similar karma. Also, specific groups within each realm share karma. In the human realm, some countries are rich, some poor, some governed well, some poorly. Certain places are devastated by conditions of war, sickness, and hunger; others flourish as oases of wealth and pleasure.

Within each group, individuals have their own karma, which has a greater influence on their experience than does collective karma. All the residents of a war-torn country share the karma of the conditions of war, yet not everyone perishes. Similarly, in a nationwide epidemic, only some will die.

In terms of the Tibetans' group karma during the Chinese invasion, some escaped the great suffering inflicted on the country as a whole, whereas others were imprisoned, tortured, or starved and endured the agony of witnessing the destruction of their country. Different people experienced different degrees of suffering.

Although the tragedy of Tibet is ongoing, it has a positive side. Because so many lamas have fled, the seedpod has broken open and the Buddhist teachings have spread throughout the world. Negative karma plays out, but so does positive karma.

When I returned to Tibet in 1987 for the first time since my escape, I went to see Tulku Arik, one of my teachers. As soon as I arrived, he asked, "Why did you leave Tibet?"

I replied, "I was sure I'd get killed."

He said, "If that hadn't been your karma, you certainly wouldn't have been killed."

My monastery, Chagdud Gonpa, still stands. Nothing was destroyed, nothing taken away. Although almost all of the surrounding monasteries were ruined, mine was untouched. Of the lamas there, one died of natural causes and another, who was politically outspoken, was imprisoned for seven years. Yet another one, a great meditator, spent a day in jail before being released. He still teaches at the monastery.

BEN: But what about the karma of those who fought to save Tibet?

RINPOCHE: It is hard to say, because you can't see inside others' minds. Did they fight because they had attachment to their own people and homeland, hatred for the Chinese, and aversion to losing their country and culture? Or did they have the understanding of a bodhisattva—that unless they stopped the Chinese from killing Tibetans, the aggressors would make terrible karma? If they were fighting with attachment and aversion, yet were motivated to save their own people, they created some benefit. But it was tainted by their hatred of the Chinese.

DARYL: When we encounter injustice, shouldn't we do something so the perpetrators don't continue to cause so much suffering? Would punishing them result in negative karma?

RINPOCHE: In some cases, punishment may help the perpetrators, though we have to be very careful that our motivation isn't stained with anger toward them or attachment to the victims. In other cases, punishment won't benefit anyone.

In Dehra Dun, India, a town populated by Tibetan refugees, we tried to build a school. The Indian government gave financial support and provided a contractor. The three-story building was expensive but went up very quickly. The day before we opened the doors, the whole structure collapsed. We found out that the builders had used cement of very poor quality.

At that point, there wasn't much to do. We had raised a lot of money to pay for the school, but no matter how much we pushed, we weren't going to get it back or the schoolhouse built. The contractor and the builders had worked very hard, and they hadn't made much money. Those of us who founded the school weren't to blame, nor was it the government's fault.

You could say it was the contractor's fault, but he didn't have enough money to pay us back. There would have been no point in suing him. We'd already lost so much, and a lawsuit would have cost us even more. It wouldn't have done us any good to send the contractor to jail; we would only have made his wife and children suffer. Ultimately, it was just our own bad karma. We wouldn't have been able to rebuild the schoolhouse by fighting or blaming someone else.

We always need to consider what will be of greatest benefit to everyone concerned. In this instance, we decided to let the whole thing go. I'm not saying that you should deal with every situation in this way. But if there is nothing to be done, drop the issue; otherwise, you will only create greater difficulties and more suffering.

DARYL: What can we do to help people who keep making negative karma?

RINPOCHE: All you can do is show them that they have other options. But don't act with resentment, self-righteousness, or condescension; you will just invite animosity and anger. Beyond that, you can pray constantly for all beings who suffer or die, as well as for those who inflict suffering. Also, pray that you will eventually be capable of completely dispelling the darkness of samsara.

HELEN: Sometimes it's difficult to tell if we're really making a difference. I've tried to help my niece, who has been suicidal on and off for ten years, but I see no change. A friend of mine, whose husband is an alcoholic, sometimes drives him places when he's drunk, to protect him and others. But perhaps she is just creating nonvirtue by enabling him. How do we know if we're really helping?

RINPOCHE: If you can help someone realize the importance of reducing mind's poisons, realizing mind's true nature, and attaining ultimate freedom, you've done something wonderful. Anything less than that is a short-term fix.

Nonetheless, something is better than nothing. If you can't help someone come to this understanding, at least you can make sure he's not going hungry. It might seem that the woman who drove her husband around just facilitated his alcoholism, but you can't assume that. She may have saved many lives.

You've helped your niece for ten years. All your efforts may seem to have been useless, but perhaps you saved her life many times over. In the process, you created virtue. The purity of your intention, not the magnitude of the results, determines how much virtue you make.

If you are condescending toward your niece, thinking that without your help she'd be lost, your virtue will be compromised. On the other hand, don't hold back until you're perfect! An offer of help made with mixed motivation is better than nothing at all. Extend yourself to others as best you can, in whatever way you can, trying to reduce your poisons as you go.

SARAH: Can the karma that leads to being hurt by an aggressor ever be avoided?

RINPOCHE: Unless it's been purified, it's unavoidable.

ALEXANDRA: I've heard that you have helped people who were physically ill. How were you able to do that if it was their karma to be sick?

RINPOCHE: If a piece of fruit is so ripe that it's about to fall off the tree, nothing can prevent it from doing so. However, if it's not ripe, a change in conditions—weather, moisture, soil—could prolong its time on the tree. A sick person's karma includes the original cause as well as the ripening conditions. Depending on his karma, a change in conditions, such as the intervention of a healer, can alter the course of his illness. If the karma to die hasn't ripened, a healer can help him buy enough time to uproot the cause of the illness through spiritual practice. Usually, for healing to take place, a person must be receptive to and have a measure of faith in the healer and the methods he uses.

Great benefit results when a spiritual practitioner purely dedicates the merit of her practice to the relief of a person's suffering. Once, a man asked me to pray for his brother, who was going to have a tumor removed. It was the biggest tumor the doctor had ever seen. I prayed for this man every day for weeks, and by the time he had surgery, the tumor had shrunk so much that it was removed without complications.

~

CONTEMPLATING CAUSE AND EFFECT

Reflecting on our day, were there missed opportunities, inwardly or outwardly, for bringing benefit to those around us? Were there missed opportunities for avoiding harm? Were there instances where we could have been more aware that those around us, whether human or animal, wanted ease, comfort, and happiness as much as we, and, just like us, wanted to avoid suffering and death? Can we see how the consequences of our awareness or confusion and inner and outer choices have unfolded in the short term? In the longer term? Then we let the mind rest.

Generating compassion for ourselves and all beings who perpetuate the causes of suffering in the very quest for happiness, we then let the mind rest.

Committing to stop the cycle, to stop creating such causes, and to purify the seeds we've already planted, again we let the mind rest.

Then we pray, for example, that we can uphold our commitment for the benefit of all beings, and let the mind rest.

16

Purifying Karma

AS WE CONTEMPLATE our past conduct, as well as the difficulty of abandoning the ten nonvirtues and practicing the ten virtues, our situation may appear to be hopeless. However, we need to remind ourselves that we can purify our karma and make different choices from now on that will affect our future.

During the time of the Buddha, there lived a man who received teachings from a charlatan. He was told that, to attain enlightenment, he had to kill a thousand people. So the man very diligently killed 999. He took a thumb from each victim and wore the thumbs as a garland around his neck.

By this time, nobody would go anywhere near him except his old mother. One day, unable to find his thousandth victim, he finally turned on her. She realized she was in great danger. Remembering that the omniscient, compassionate Buddha would aid anyone who called on him, she prayed fervently. He immediately appeared between her and her son.

The son was delighted that the Buddha had shown up, because now he wouldn't have to kill his mother; he could kill the Buddha instead. But each time he tried to attack him, the Buddha appeared farther away. With every step forward that the man took, the Buddha seemed even more distant. Going after the

Buddha was like trying to catch a rainbow. Finally, the man stopped and asked him, "How do you do that?"

The Buddha replied, "I am enlightened. I have no karma, so you can't harm me. You have been terribly misled. Killing people will not liberate you from suffering—it will send you to hell. If you want to attain enlightenment, you must purify your karma."

The Buddha then taught the man how to go about such purification. He explained the value of being virtuous and accumulating merit and wisdom. The man changed his conduct, practiced extensive purification, and in that very lifetime became an *arhat,* one who has refined away all karma and mental poisons.

No mistake or misdeed is so great that it cannot be purified. For generations, Tibetans have been inspired by the life story of the great saint Milarepa. His father died when he was just a child, and thereafter his mother, sister, and he suffered great hardship at the hands of his uncle and aunt. To please his vindictive mother, he became skilled in black magic and caused the tragic deaths of a number of people and animals. When at length he understood the gravity of what he had done, he gave up his wicked ways to become a Buddhist practitioner. In his lifetime, he purified all of his karma, attained great realization and, finally, enlightenment. Even now, when people read his story or even hear his name, they are motivated to turn toward the spiritual path.

In a former lifetime, the great lama Dodrubchen Rinpoche was a horse thief who robbed the inhabitants of one region on behalf of his own people. During one of his raids, he stole a pregnant mare. As he made his escape, she was unable to keep up with the other horses and lay down.

The thief was furious at the thought that the owners might get their horse back, along with the colt she was carrying. Drawing his sword, he sliced open the mare's body, and the colt fell out. As she lay dying, the mother lifted her head to look at her baby. When he saw the mare's love, the thief was filled with great remorse and vowed from that time forward never to hurt another being.

Having decided to take up a life of spiritual practice, he sold his horse and weapons, bought some tea, and set out on a pilgrimage to central Tibet, where he hoped to receive teachings from the renowned master Jigmé Lingpa. Upon arriving in Lhasa, he made arrangements to sell the tea and use the money as an offering, but discovered that the tea was gone. The horse thief had himself been robbed and had nothing to offer the master. Nonetheless, he was given the teachings and in that lifetime gained mastery over his mind.

Though the potency of negative karma cannot be denied, such karma can be purified by the practice of compassion as well as formal meditation techniques. One method involves the four powers of purification, which parallel the four steps leading to full karmic consequences: the object, intention, action, and consequences.

The first is the power of support. We visualize in front of us a manifestation of wisdom from our spiritual tradition—for example, Buddha, God, Jesus, Tara, or Vajrasattva—as the witness to our purification.

The second involves acknowledging and taking responsibility for what we have done, making no excuses. In the presence of the wisdom being, we confess and express deep regret for all of our harmful actions of body, speech, and mind, whether intentional or inadvertent, remembered or forgotten, both in this and countless past lives. Because we have accumulated a vast store of negativity with tragic karmic consequences, our regret must be genuine. We should feel it as intensely as if we had carelessly drunk a bottle of water only to discover that it was laced with arsenic.

The third power is our resolve not to repeat what we have done. We understand that actions motivated by anger, attachment, ignorance, pride, or jealousy will have serious repercussions, so our commitment to uprooting those poisons and refraining from such actions must be wholehearted. We cannot try to purify our harmful acts in a superficial way, thinking that if we repeat them, we can simply purify them again. Rather, we must sincerely commit ourselves to turning away, once and for all, from the causes of suffering.

The fourth power is the actual purification. The wisdom being responds to our regret and commitment with an outpouring of love and compassion in the form of light or nectar that washes through us, completely purifying our karma.

It is said that the only virtue of nonvirtue is that it can be purified. By repeatedly relying on these four powers, we can purify the negativity we have created in this and previous lifetimes. As mental poisons arise and we commit more harmful actions, we continue to purify them until not even the propensity to harm remains. We eliminate not just the temporary conditions of suffering, but its very cause.

It is important to purify karma daily. There is rarely, if ever, a day when we do not cause harm in some way. Before we go to bed at night, we might think, "This could be the last day of my life. Once I fall asleep, I may not wake up again. I have heard of strong, young people dying in their sleep. This could be my last moment of consciousness. What have I done with my life? Have I helped others, or have I hurt them with my actions, words, and thoughts? If I live through the night, I resolve to change my behavior, to help rather than harm."

Then we look back on the day and recall the moments when we couldn't hold our tongue, when we gave in to jealousy or a nasty thought. Regretting our mistakes and our lack of control, we purify them using the four powers.

Next we recall our virtuous actions and, instead of feeling proud, dedicate the merit, freely offering all the virtue we have ever accumulated in this and past lifetimes and all we will create in the future. We pray that, by this merit, the causes of suffering for all beings will be eliminated and all may realize their perfect nature. To the extent that we do this, our own mind will become pure. To the extent that our mind is pure, we will be able to benefit others.

Although we aspire to purify our karma before it manifests, purification is inherent in the ripening process itself. Through our current suffering, we repay part or all of our karmic debt. We might think that as spiritual practitioners we should be free of misery. But sickness, including a long chronic illness, or a slow painful death can exhaust karma that would otherwise result in suffering for eons in the lower realms. The longer we live, the greater our opportunity for purification. This is why suicide and mercy killing amount to tragic wastes.

Once, a woman with cancer came to see me. Her face was grotesque—so enlarged that her eyes had been pushed to either side of her head. She wore a button that said, "Don't ask." She said that when children looked at her, unable to control their horror, they would scream and run away. I told her that whenever someone was repulsed by her, some of her karma was purified. I also said that I had great respect for her and considered her a bodhisattva, because no adult who saw her could help but feel compassion and appreciate his own good fortune. I told her not to be discouraged; by her extreme suffering, she was purifying the dregs of her negative karma. The worst of our karma sometimes ripens just before our liberation.

At one time, I knew a genuine renunciate who didn't have a family or home and didn't care about money. He lived very simply in the woods. At the end of his life, he was hospitalized with throat cancer. A lama offered him an empowerment, or initiation, into a practice that would aid him as he died. He declined, saying, "I may be sick now, but this is the last of my karma ripening, and then I will be free."

Unless we have the omniscience of a buddha, we cannot know for certain the trajectory of someone's karma. Although one person's life may be very difficult, he is purifying karma. Someone else's circumstances may seem fortunate on the surface, but he may actually be in a downward spiral.

Once there was a yogi practicing in a cave, and in another one nearby lived a nun who was a very good practitioner. With his clairvoyance, the yogi could see that the nun would be reborn as a *dri,* a female yak. He thought, "How strange! How could such an excellent practitioner be reborn as a pack animal?" Then he looked out at a hawk perched in a tree and saw that it would take rebirth as a beautiful boy who would hold a powerful spiritual position.

The yogi was surprised by this seeming paradox—that someone so virtuous could be reborn as a pack animal, whereas a bird so predatory could be reborn as an exalted human. Looking more closely, he saw that the nun had purified all but the remnants of her negative karma, which would produce rebirth as a dri. Once she had purified that karma, she would be liberated and return to the human realm, not by the force of karma, but only to benefit beings. However, the boy, though regarded as an inspiration to spiritual practitioners, would be reborn in a hell realm for having deceived his followers and misused his spiritual authority.

Purifying karma is like trying to wear down an iron pillar with a fingernail file or leveling a great mountain using a teaspoon. One daily meditation session isn't sufficient to refine away the huge amount of karma we've accumulated. After having meditated for a while, we might wonder if we are doing something wrong. Spiritual practice is supposed to eliminate suffering, yet we keep getting sick, and meditation makes our body ache. But we have to do more than a teaspoon's worth of practice a day.

Purification takes patience, diligence, and perseverance. During this painstaking process, we may not experience big changes all at once, but as we gradually refine away our obscurations, like removing a blindfold, we will come to perceive mind's nature.

In our suffering, mistakes, and negative emotions lies the potential for transformation. If we slipped and fell off a cliff, breaking all our bones, we would know never to walk along the edge of the cliff again. The path to enlightenment is fraught with difficulties and challenges, but if we can learn from our experiences, our progress will be swifter. To make flour, we need stones to grind the grain. If we expect the wind to accomplish this task, we will have to wait a long time. Our pain and anguish are like grinding stones that can help us refine away our obscurations.

TERESA: When we practice purification using the four powers, do we actually bring to mind each harmful act we've committed?

RINPOCHE: If it helps you to develop genuine remorse, you can try to recall your harmful actions, although you won't remember them all. And even if you could, it would take you a long, long time to review your life. So recall your worst actions, knowing that there are many others you've forgotten. You have created oceans of nonvirtue; generate great regret for all of it.

VINCENT: If you've consciously or unconsciously hurt someone, is an apology a part of the purification process?

RINPOCHE: From a spiritual perspective, when you sincerely regret and purify what you've done to someone, the karma is finished. But if you know that things are still unresolved for the other person, you can try to put her at ease. You have to be careful, though, because if she responds negatively, she might rekindle your anger, reopen the wound, and make the situation worse. Why go through it all again? Your desire to engage her arises because you haven't reached your own resolution. Don't make her jump through hoops for your own comfort. If you have personally resolved the situation and are treating her with love and compassion, the conflict will probably exhaust itself.

VINCENT: How is our karma actually purified through spiritual practice?

RINPOCHE: To cut a diamond, you use a diamond; to cut iron, you use iron. When your mind has made a mistake, you use the power of mind to purify that mistake.

ALEXANDRA: I've recited some purification mantras and tried to act more carefully but still find myself reinforcing the patterns I want to transform. It seems that my practice isn't working very well.

RINPOCHE: We've accumulated karma for eons, so our purification practice can't be feeble, superficial, or insincere. We must wholeheartedly regret our harmful actions, not because we're ashamed or embarrassed about them or don't want to suffer in the future, but because we recognize that, like us, all beings are caught in a web of confusion and negative karma. Our compassion for them inspires us to deepen our practice. Without making a profound commitment to practice, we won't be able to overcome the force of our past karma.

Not long ago, there lived a very powerful Tibetan who had killed many men and animals. He was an excellent marksman who could shoot even the elusive musk deer without getting off his horse. Although he lived in a country where Buddhism thrived, he didn't do any spiritual practice. Still, he knew that his days were numbered and that, because of his actions, he would be in big trouble when he died. So he went to a great lama and asked what his next rebirth would be.

The lama replied, "I'm not sure, but between the two of us we can find out. If we both strongly pray, something is sure to become clear."

The man had some faith, so he prayed fervently before going to bed. That night, he dreamt that he was old and sick. Many lamas and doctors tried to help him, to no avail, and his life slipped away. He immediately took rebirth in a hell realm, where he endured great torment.

After eons in hell, he was born as a wolf. One day, he came upon a Mani wall—a wall of stones on which millions of *Om Mani Padme Hung* mantras had been carved. In his past life as the hunter, the wall had been too high for a man sitting on a horse to reach. Now it had eroded to half his height, so he knew that he had been in hell for a long time.

Then the hunter woke up, extremely shaken. He ran to the lama crying, filled with remorse for everything he had done. He vowed that he would never kill another person or animal. The lama said, "It is very good to make that vow, but your murderous habit remains strong. A hundred more men will die by your hand."

The hunter was in despair. He had killed a lot of people, but certainly not a hundred, and he couldn't bear to think of killing so many more. He stopped hunting and gave the lama half of his wealth, asking that he use it to create virtue by offering it to a monastery or buying food for the poor.

Not long after that, the man and a group of his powerful friends, all wealthy merchants, traveled to a far-off country to purchase goods. On their way home, thieves overtook them and threatened to take everything they had. Before the man's companions could defend themselves, he said to them, "I know that you can easily kill these brigands, but don't do it. Let them have everything. When we get home, I will replace your losses. I don't want to kill anymore."

His friends protested that surrendering to the thieves would be shameful. "Don't worry," the man replied. "People will think that we were generous, not cowardly. They will realize that we could have killed these thieves."

Because his friends trusted him, they agreed to do things his way. When the thieves again demanded their goods, the man said to them, "You have heard of me and my strength. You know how easily I could kill you. But I'm not going to; I will let you have everything. Remember this act of kindness. Don't forget that I didn't kill you today."

One of the thieves pointed a gun at the man and said contemptuously, "Who the hell are you?" Then he slapped him in the face. In that moment, the man's generous and compassionate intentions vanished. He grabbed the gun and turned it on the thieves, killing four of them. His remorse wasn't sufficient to overcome his karmic pattern of killing.

DARYL: Is there anything we can do to purify someone else's karma?

RINPOCHE: Karma can be purified only by the person who made it. But since one of the causes of suffering is a lack of merit, you can help someone by creating merit and dedicating it to her.

IMANI: I feel uncomfortable basing my actions on the motivation of reward or punishment. Can I take a wider perspective, such as the view that everything is empty? I want the students at our university to develop their own sense of right and wrong, not to act positively only because they fear punishment or desire a reward.

RINPOCHE: Imagine going to a doctor, saying, "I don't want to hear about illness or medicine. I just want to be healthy." The loftier view you refer to is certainly taught in the Buddhist tradition, but if you want to get to the rooftop, you have to take the staircase. You have to go through a process of thoroughly assimilating the teachings point by point to arrive at genuine realization of mind's nature.

To untangle a ball of knotted chains in your jewelry box, you first have to untie the outermost one. Then you work on the next, and continue from there. We may appreciate the simplicity of our true nature, but it is concealed beneath a mass of knots. To get to it, we must untie them one by one.

∾

PURIFICATION THROUGH COMPASSION

We practice the "Developing Compassion" meditation (p. 87) earnestly and as often as possible, so that the urgent wish and commitment to alleviate all pain and misery arise spontaneously and pervasively, whether or not we are directly encountering suffering.

Throughout the day we draw on this compassion, our heart never separate from the needs of others. We make our compassion and commitment to end all suffering the basis not only of every meditation but, as well, of every action, word, or thought throughout our lives, until this motivation completely pervades our experience. The more fully our compassion permeates our lives, the more quickly we are able to purify past actions and accumulate merit, swiftly increasing the spontaneous presence of bodhicitta, the awakened mind.

THE FOUR POWERS OF PURIFICATION

These four steps or powers of purification, the means by which we can purify and transform negative habits and impulses, are undertaken sequentially. We begin by relying on the first power—that of support or witness, the reflection of our inherent purity—by visualizing, above and in front of us, whosoever or whatsoever embodies for us limitless wisdom, compassion, and capacity to benefit.

The second power involves honestly, sincerely, and profoundly regretting all the harm we have ever created with body, speech, and mind, whether forgotten or remembered, in this or past lives. We can reflect on recent or distant actions we're conscious of, the magnitude of those unconsciously undertaken, or both.

The third power involves our resolution, our firm commitment, never, under any circumstances, to repeat such actions, and to use our spiritual tools to change the habits that have led to these actions.

We then envision radiant light flowing to us from the support or witness to our purification, infusing us with the blessing of the illumination of that inherent purity, as all of our nonvirtue and obscurations are purified through this fourth power.

Ideally, we try to practice the four powers during the day whenever we think, say, or do something that we regret, and every night as we review the day before going to sleep.

PART III

The Path of Change

17

The Six Perfections

THE FOUR IMMEASURABLE QUALITIES of equanimity, compassion, love, and rejoicing are the cornerstones of bodhicitta, the very foundation of pure-hearted motivation. The development of bodhicitta involves three steps. First by cultivating the four immeasurable qualities, we give rise to bodhicitta. Second, we establish enlightenment—our own and that of all beings—as our goal; this is wishing bodhicitta. Our aspiration is based on the realization that anything short of enlightenment is of only temporary benefit. Thorough contemplation of the four thoughts brings us to the unshakable conviction that, unless we awaken from this dream, the cycles of suffering will go on endlessly.

But aspiration is not enough. We need to do whatever we can, through service and spiritual practice, to benefit others temporarily and ultimately. To do so skillfully and effectively, we train in the six perfections. This practice provides an extremely effective framework for undertaking the third step—engaging bodhicitta—in which we apply the methods that enable us to accomplish our goal.

The firm resolve of bodhicitta, made with pure heart, and selfless dedication of merit, sets in motion a momentum that never ceases to produce virtue and benefit until liberation. The power of this resolution is such that the virtue created is as vast as the sky. Having awakened bodhicitta in our heart, we embark irrevocably on the path to enlightenment; nothing could prevent us from reaching our destination.

GENEROSITY

The first of the six perfections, generosity—offering our time, effort, and resources—is an excellent means of accumulating merit and increasing virtuous qualities. Generosity counteracts miserliness and self-clinging. As we learn that we always have something to give, if only a kind word, we allay our fear of deprivation and avert the karmic consequences of greed, craving, dissatisfaction, selfishness, and hoarding. Moreover, we loosen our attachment and create conditions for our own and others' happiness and ultimate well-being. When we dedicate the merit, our generosity extends even further, to all beings in every realm. Over time on the bodhisattva path, we cease to value ourselves above others—we give away our self-cherishing.

Our present good fortune is not an accident, but the fruit of previous generosity. We take advantage of our positive circumstances by giving, thus planting more virtuous seeds and accumulating the merit we need to continue benefiting others in the future.

There are three kinds of generosity. First, the generosity of substance, involves freely giving money and material possessions without concern for compensation or reciprocation. We don't need great wealth, only a generous spirit. Rather than tossing our leftovers in the garbage, we can put them in a place where animals can find them. We won't lose anything by doing so;

think how happy we would be if we were hungry and someone fed us. Or we might carry someone's heavy bag, help another onto a bus, or bring cheer to a friend having a bad day by telling a funny story. Just as water fills a bucket drop by drop, no act of generosity is insignificant, no offering too small.

Once, during a procession, the Buddha passed a young boy eating some beans. Moved by the sight of the Buddha, the boy cast a few toward him as an offering. Three of them hit the Buddha's heart and four fell into his bowl. The merit of having given only seven beans was sufficient for the boy to enjoy great riches and power for many lifetimes.

The extent of our selflessness and the purity of our motivation, as well as the recipient of our offering, determine the merit we create. Giving a glass of water to a thirsty person with the motivation of bodhicitta, followed by sincere dedication, produces incalculably more merit than doing so without such motivation. Offering water to someone who is not thirsty produces less, while offering it to our object of faith results in the most merit.

The second kind of generosity is that of communication. This includes guiding or consoling someone and sharing spiritual teachings, which produces even greater merit than the generosity of substance.

Even if we aren't qualified or authorized to teach others, we can suggest a helpful book or a workshop being given by a reputable teacher. We can offer an example of selflessness, or we can share personal experiences that illustrate the value of virtuous thoughts and actions. One of the greatest gifts is having a positive impact on someone's mind. By helping people understand the repercussions of harmful versus beneficial actions, we help them take some control over their future.

The third kind of generosity is protecting those who are afraid, including those whose lives may be in jeopardy. We might shield a battered woman from her husband's abuse, as well as prevent the husband from suffering the terrible consequences of continuing to beat her. Or we might give the gift of life to humans and animals through our efforts to preserve the environment. Ultimately, by guiding others toward enlightenment, we protect them from the suffering of samsara.

We need to take every opportunity to practice generosity. We don't have to pick a rose from a bush to offer it to someone. We can offer in our imagination anything that gives us pleasure. If we come across a pure mountain stream, rather than thinking, "I wish this were on my land," or "Why can't we have this in Los Angeles?" we rejoice that such pure water exists and offer it to our object of faith. As we stroll through someone's garden or beautiful home, rather than thinking, "I wish all this wealth and beauty were mine!" we can offer it as well.

MORAL DISCIPLINE

Moral discipline, the second of the six perfections, has three aspects. The first consists of reducing our harmful thoughts, words, and actions. The second includes creating virtue and dedicating the merit to all beings. The third involves making an unstinting effort to be of greater benefit through the skillful use of body, speech, and mind.

Moral discipline is not a matter of correcting others, but of disciplining ourselves. Some people think that moral discipline is required only of monks and nuns, entailing vows of celibacy, abstinence from alcohol or meat, and so forth. However, we all need to be extremely scrupulous in our physical, verbal, and mental conduct, and that requires discipline. In each moment, we make a conscious choice, assessing what we are doing and why, without making excuses for ourselves. Just as we constantly adjust the steering wheel when we drive a car so we don't veer to one side of the road, we constantly adjust the mind to prevent ourselves from deviating to extremes in our thought or behavior. When we consistently ascertain whether we are acting out of selfishness or selflessness, our positive qualities will increase and endure, and our negative habits will diminish and fall away. We will develop even greater discernment as we continue on the path.

In a larger sense, moral discipline involves abandoning mind's poisons, maintaining good heart, and continually expanding our motivation to include all beings in the embrace of our thoughts and aspirations.

Because we often unwittingly harm others, not only physically but also verbally, we must always be mindful. Words are very powerful and can cause great injury. Rather than speaking out immediately, we need to think carefully about what we want to say. Even though we may not harm anyone with our body or speech, if in our mind we have the intention to harm others, or rejoice in their misfortune, we will still create negative karma.

Moral discipline also involves doing everything possible to create virtue, developing useful skills or conditions to support our endeavors. This means being responsive to the needs of others, explaining ourselves clearly in terms they can comprehend, and being sensitive to their culture or religion, as well as their receptivity. When someone is tired of listening or resistant to what we have to say, we should stop talking. People will reject what is imposed on them.

Finally, moral discipline involves unsparing effort to help others. If there is anything we can do, we act selflessly without holding back, never claiming we're too tired or busy or that what we're doing is more important than coming to someone's aid. If we perfect moral discipline, we can benefit anyone who sees, hears, touches, or remembers us.

PATIENCE

The third perfection, patience, is our great friend because it helps us overcome anger, the most powerful form of nonvirtue. The first of three kinds of patience is forbearance in the face of personal difficulty or adversity—enduring harm, negativity, or abuse without becoming angry or retaliating. We need to practice patience with everyone in our life, understanding that they, like us, are subject to mind's poisons. We must learn to respond to them calmly rather than in the usual impulsive way.

Being patient is difficult enough when things go wrong, but is even more challenging when everyone seems to be reacting negatively. Although there is virtue in refraining from openly expressing anger, true patience means that anger isn't even present in the mind. Appearing outwardly patient while stewing on the inside, holding resentment, will only make everything worse in time.

Negativity that arises in our mind in response to conflict is as much an obstacle as is outer difficulty. Like a series of dominoes falling, discord among people creates more conflict, which in turn creates more negativity, and so on. The truth is that there will always be problems in any group: many holy statues carried in a bag are going to clink against each other.

From the perspective of a bodhisattva, obstacles and enemies give us a chance to practice. If we were happy all the time, there would be no opportunity to develop forbearance. Instead of backing away from adversity, trying to avoid problems or deflect negativity directed toward us, we can use whatever arises to strengthen our patience. In this way, those who harm us become our benefactors.

We patiently work things through, solving problems as we go. We not only learn to accept our difficulties, but pray that by our suffering, the suffering of all other beings may cease. With acceptance and compassion, we can develop the patience necessary to continue helping others even when they provoke us.

Once, Mahatma Gandhi encountered a man trying to carry three suitcases at a British railway station. Gandhi offered to help him and carried two of them. Upon arriving at the man's home, Gandhi set the suitcases down and they fell over. The man was so upset that he slapped Gandhi. Gandhi didn't respond. When the man opened his bag to pay him, Gandhi explained that he had helped him not in hope of payment, but because he saw him struggling. Hearing this, the man felt tremendous regret.

The second kind of patience applies to spiritual practice. It is what enables us to endure the physical and emotional difficulties we sometimes face as practitioners. If we understand the importance of accumulating merit and wisdom, we won't back away and our good heart will give us the strength to be patient.

The third kind of patience enables us to confront the fear that can arise when our ordinary concepts fall away and we experience the emptiness of phenomena. The teachings on emptiness make many people afraid. They feel they have nothing to hold on to. And, indeed, we do not. When we die, no matter how much we may want to keep this body and remain with those we love, only our karma will go with us. If, in this lifetime, we stabilize our recognition of mind's true nature, we can attain liberation at the moment of death. Knowing this gives us great incentive to keep practicing, meditating patiently without fear.

DILIGENCE

The fourth perfection is diligence. Fully appreciating our opportunity as human beings, we work tirelessly and persistently to benefit ourselves and others, as well as to increase our ability to help. On the spiritual path, diligence is more important than intelligence. No matter how dull our minds or difficult our circumstances, with diligence we can accomplish our spiritual goals, progressing one step at a time, day by day, without losing ground.

Diligence is the antidote to our biggest obstacle on the path: laziness. This is not to say that we are always negligent or lax, but our enthusiasm often turns the wrong way—toward samsara. We are unstinting in pursuing our worldly desires and ambitions. But now, having embarked on a spiritual path, we must direct our energy toward purely motivated, virtuous activities.

There are three kinds of diligence. The first, armorlike diligence, involves getting a sense of the task at hand, then preparing for and making a commitment to it. Whenever necessary, we review the teachings as a reminder of why we want to help.

The second is diligence in action. We do our best in all circumstances, maintaining our pure motivation and commitment to the goal. We don't allow ourselves to be thwarted by negative habits or personal obstacles, such as anger, laziness, or procrastination, that are products of our own mind. Even if they temporarily divert our attention, we refocus, renew our commitment, and keep going. We don't ignore or deny what needs to be done. Rather than being daunted by the idea that we are working for innumerable beings, we rejoice in the opportunity to help them. Even if others laugh at or try to stop us, we don't lose our enthusiasm, but persevere. We maintain a steady pace and experience the joy of accomplishment; that way we keep from burning out. We act quickly because we know that our present circumstances are temporary. As long as we are alive, we have the opportunity to be of benefit.

For this reason, it is important to be diligent in our spiritual practice. If our meditation is going so well that we think we can walk on water, we should remind ourselves that things change. When our meditation seems unsteady, we need to remember that we have traveled a long way down the rocky road of duality, and we face a long, slow ride home to mind's nature. When our knees hurt, rather than resist or avoid the pain, we accept it, knowing that we are purifying karma. When our meditation goes well, we keep going. When it doesn't, we keep going. Whatever happens—pain or pleasure, extreme doubt or bliss—we keep moving forward.

There was once a man who had to climb a number of foothills and a very high mountain whenever he went to receive teachings from the Buddha. Every time he got to the top of one hill, it seemed that another arose before him. He invariably became very tired and discouraged. Finally, he took his problem to the Buddha, who asked, "Where do you look as you climb?"

The man replied, "I look ahead, in the direction I am going."

The Buddha replied, "Every now and then, look back to see how far you've come."

As we make the long, steep journey for the temporary and ultimate benefit of every being, we can sometimes look back at the changes that have taken place in our mind, heart, and life. Then, as we rejoice and dedicate the merit, we reaffirm our intention to persevere, staying focused on our goal in order to achieve it. We need to find the right balance between reflecting on our accomplishments when we need inspiration and concentrating on our destination when we need more diligence, and between pushing too hard in our meditation and becoming lost in distraction.

The third kind of diligence is referred to as unstoppable diligence. It arises as our practice matures and we gain confidence in our spiritual tools, together with our ability to use them to benefit others. Our counterproductive habits decrease, and our positive qualities and ability to deal with negative experiences increase, until our diligence becomes effortless and spontaneous.

CONCENTRATION

The fifth perfection is concentration, also called meditative stability. We continually bring the mind back to effortful or effortless meditation. We break down habits that perpetuate suffering and focus on methods that bring about temporary and ultimate happiness. Without concentration, even if we were to spend the rest of our life in solitary retreat, our mind would wander endlessly—dancing in and out of attachment, aversion, pride, and jealousy, hope and fear, good and bad—and we would never be able to help anyone. A genuine ability to benefit doesn't result from trying to figure out the universe, but from changing the mind, using methods that will enable us to relax into the openness of our true nature.

Becoming attached to temporary meditative experiences of bliss, clarity, and stability characterizes what is called childlike concentration. Becoming attached to the experience of emptiness is often referred to as clear concentration. Finally, what is called the excellent concentration of the buddhas arises when, free of all attachment, we rest in unwavering recognition of mind's nature.

As beginning practitioners, we concentrate on distinguishing between virtue and nonvirtue. As we become aware of the predominance of nonvirtue in our mind, we learn to turn away from negativity. Focusing repeatedly on virtue, we develop wholesome habits of body, speech, and mind. Finally, we come to rest effortlessly in recognition of our true nature, and this becomes our main practice. We realize that phenomena appear like rainbows or clouds—or like the rising and setting of the moon and sun—in the vastness of the sky, which itself never changes. We rest with clarity and awareness in the skylike nature of mind.

WISDOM

Having cultivated the three kinds of wisdom, which come from listening to, contemplating, and meditating on spiritual teachings, we investigate phenomena to ascertain whether they are permanent, singular, or free of outside influences—the three criteria by which something is determined to be absolutely true. Although we tend to assume that things are stable—even permanent—they all change. Everything is composite, created by causes and conditions, and made up of elements that have joined together and can come apart. Finally, nothing is free; everything we hold to as real can be affected or destroyed by outer or inner influences.

The body, for example, is not permanent. At one time it did not exist, and sooner or later it will cease to be. It is not singular but a combination of many things: flesh, blood, bones, and so on. If we examine each of these down to the level of subatomic particles, we find nothing at all. Finally, the body is not free. It can be affected by other things.

The fact that phenomena are apparent yet not ultimately true leads us to the meaning of the true nature of reality, beyond the extremes of existence and nonexistence. Even as phenomena occur, their nature is emptiness. This is what the Buddha meant when he said, "Form is emptiness. Emptiness is form. Form is none other than emptiness. Emptiness is none other than form." The display of phenomena arises simultaneously with emptiness. As in a dream, though appearances manifest, nothing actually comes into being and nothing actually ceases. Nothing really comes or goes. Phenomena cannot be said to be one, yet in that their true nature is the same absolute truth, neither are they many.

Explanations such as this can help us come to a conceptual understanding of the nature of mind. But that nature lies beyond words and concepts, so we can experience it directly only through nondual wisdom. This is the sixth perfection, *prajnaparamita*, the perfection of wisdom, or great knowing. Beyond this, there is no goal.

We practice the first five perfections to cultivate and express bodhicitta in the context of our dream reality, the relative truth. By applying the sixth perfection of great knowing to our practice of the other five, we bring an extraordinary quality to our activities. Ordinary generosity becomes the perfection of generosity—generosity sealed with great knowing—when we know that there is no inherent truth to the giver, the recipient, or the interaction between them. If we recognize the true nature of our action beyond the three spheres, we will neither feel attachment to it, nor deny that it is taking place on the relative level. The more we cultivate great knowing, the more we can liberate the poisons of the mind. We will begin to see things differently, to deal more calmly with everything that arises, and to be of greater benefit.

Although we have discussed the six perfections as distinct qualities, they are most effective if applied together. For example, ideally when we engage in spiritual practice, we are motivated by generosity in our intention to benefit others. We apply moral discipline by being careful not to make mistakes. However difficult our meditation, we persevere with patience and diligence. We apply concentration, at the same time recognizing our true nature.

These days, some practitioners prefer to emphasize the absolute truth, placing less value on practicing the first five perfections. But we are trapped by our belief in the relative truth. So until we have attained full realization, we need to carefully apply all six to every action, relying on relative methods to cut our delusion. If we are tied up with rope, no amount of talking about its empty nature will loosen it. Until our mind breaks free of duality, we will remain fettered by relative truth.

In the very act of dreaming this existence, we perpetuate the dream by responding to what we believe is true. Until our actions are imbued with wisdom, we will never awaken altogether.

Because of their wisdom, bodhisattvas do not invest relative appearances with solidity and are therefore able to practice the six perfections flawlessly. No longer subject to false assumptions about reality, they can work unstintingly, patiently, and carefully for others, realizing that in a dream body they are making dream efforts to do whatever is necessary for dream beings. Free of attachment and aversion, their efforts to benefit others are unhampered. They work without self-clinging and fear of loss because they know that, ultimately, nothing in this world can truly be gained or lost. They function within the dream without being invested in it; they are in the world but not of it.

Just as a bird needs two wings to fly, we need to accumulate both merit and wisdom. Through our practice of the six perfections, we accumulate merit in the context of relative truth and wisdom in the context of absolute truth. This leads to the two types of benefit—enlightenment for oneself and unceasing benefit for others.

PRACTICING THE SIX PERFECTIONS
IN RELATIONSHIPS

Relationships offer a wealth of opportunity for practicing the six perfections. When we interact with others selflessly, our altruism embodies generosity. Generously expressing our love through body, speech, and mind, exploring ways to please, and helping others find fulfillment form the foundation for joyful and successful relationships.

We practice moral discipline by living according to our spiritual principles and emphasizing positive qualities such as loving kindness and virtue. We eliminate selfish, petty, and irritating habits that upset others, and refrain from careless actions that might cause harm or unhappiness. We focus on one another's needs, and rather than holding on to fixed ideas about how relationships should be and insisting that others change, we work on our own flaws.

Patience is pivotal to successful relationships. It is rooted in a commitment to maintaining harmony regardless of any external or emotional changes our loved ones undergo. Arguing wastes time, and self-righteousness only perpetuates suffering. If we stay patient, disagreements are more likely to resolve.

Upholding a commitment to any relationship, and to mutual benefit within it, requires diligence and unflagging effort. We develop these qualities by focusing on the bond between us rather than on our problems and by being prepared to meet obstacles with courage. Many challenges will test our commitment, but we must nevertheless persevere. What is important is not what arises in the course of our lives together, but how we respond in each situation to ensure that our relationships and practice endure.

Learning what brings happiness to ourselves and others, as well as remaining mindful of our interactions, requires concentration. When problems occur, we need to remember that everything that comes together eventually falls apart. Then we won't focus on what will not last, such as youthful attractiveness, but rather on the causes of temporary and ultimate benefit.

Finally, we must recognize that all we experience in our relationships—joy, sorrow, everyday events, and moments of high drama—is impermanent, like a dream, a magical illusion, or a mirage. This perspective will reduce the common causes of strife: attachment to things going our way and aversion to difficulties. We bring balance to our relationships by remembering that it is our reactions to outer conditions, not the conditions themselves, that cause happiness and unhappiness. If we maintain this view as well as pure motivation, our relationships will produce happiness in this and future lives, and embody the essence of the spiritual path.

As we apply the six perfections to our interactions with those close to us, and expand outwardly from there, our relationships begin to transform. Not only do we ourselves change, but our kindness, patience, and compassion touch the lives of everyone around us.

ANGELA: When you spoke about generosity, you said we could offer a beautiful house that we happen to see. How can I offer something I don't own?

RINPOCHE: All appearances are projections of our mind. In that sense, we're co-owners of whatever arises. By virtue of shared karma, all beings are co-creators of this universe. So we can give what we have a part in, even though it may not literally belong to us. We can be very generous with the entire universe.

IMANI: Being generous with my time, that's my issue! I struggle with how to be kind to my students and fellow faculty members without getting used up. Many students need help, but there is no way I can help them all and still keep body and mind intact.

RINPOCHE: Following the spiritual path means never compromising your fundamental compassion. The welfare of others is your sole concern. However, sometimes accomplishing that requires setting limits.

Decide how much you can do with pure heart. Anything beyond that might make you resentful, diminishing the virtue you have created. Generosity takes training. If it is hard for you to give and if the recipient of your gift doesn't express appreciation, you will experience regret and disappointment. Serving others without limit until nothing is left of us is an exalted path. But at first, it is an extremely difficult one to follow. So we offer what we can to the best of our ability and dedicate the merit of our efforts to all beings. This increases our ability to serve with pure motivation.

SARAH: Maybe I could share my quandary and get some feedback. I work as an aide in a mental health unit. The patients there come with a lot of mixed-up thoughts. Medication helps reduce the auditory and visual hallucinations of some of them. But those who don't respond to medication are absolutely terrified, their lives filled with pain. Often the only thing we can do is to keep them safe. We provide food and a place to sleep, and protect them from harming themselves or others. Could you suggest anything else?

RINPOCHE: Really, there isn't much more to do than provide safety, make sure their physical needs are met, and offer any kindness you can.

Sometimes the karma that results in such an illness lasts a lifetime, sometimes only a relatively short period. Certain people can go back and forth between confusion and clarity, like fish leaping in and out of water.

We can't take a direct approach to mind training with those who have mental imbalances. They seldom have a reference point we can work from. They have their own unique take on reality, their own truth, their own world experience. Sometimes an extraordinary therapist can help them begin to walk back out, but that is very rare. Usually when they try to meditate, they work too hard and go off into a corner of their mind that is even more unbalanced. They can't find a middle ground.

I attempt to help such people by suggesting they eat frequently and very well. I recommend that rather than try to meditate, they relax without too much quiet or isolation. They can perform small tasks that aren't stressful, as stress only exacerbates the imbalance. A spacious outer and inner environment with no pressure or demands and a supportive daily routine can sometimes help bring them back to a state of balance.

ALEXANDRA: The teachings on emptiness are so life-altering. Wouldn't sharing them with others be extremely generous?

RINPOCHE: It is easy to say that the nature of everything is emptiness: the nature of anger is emptiness, the nature of hope is emptiness, everything is emptiness. But if someone slaps you, it doesn't feel like emptiness. The Buddhist teachings on emptiness are very profound. We can't hope to understand them in five days, or by reading one book, or even a thousand. Just talking about them won't bring us any closer to realization of their inner meaning. We have to have a genuine and stable personal experience of emptiness before we can ever hope to share it.

I am now quite old and have spent my life studying, meditating upon, and applying these teachings. I may have some small ability to answer people's questions; even so, it's not easy to speak about something that defies concepts. If you try to explain emptiness to others, you are likely to upset their minds as well as your own. That is not the purpose of these teachings.

It takes a long time to become skillful in communicating the Buddhist teachings to others. Impermanence is a good place to start because people can see it everywhere. Discussing movies and television—how writers, directors, and actors create elaborate illusions that we invest with reality, responding with excitement, laughter, and tears—is also a way of demonstrating how phenomena arise from mind.

One approach won't work for everyone. If a person can't relate to your view, you won't be able to help. For example, framing someone's experience in terms of karma will be ineffective if she doesn't understand or agree with that principle. You might instead point out how negative actions breed more negativity and suffering. If you develop a genuine understanding of karma and other spiritual truths, you can facilitate others' understanding, no matter what their backgrounds.

In terms of sharing what you've learned here, when you are asked, speak from your own experience. But be honest about what you don't know. If you integrate these teachings into your life, your actions will have far more impact on others' minds than anything you could put into words. Anyone can give lectures, but how you live has much greater value.

SARAH: I'm only nineteen and feel a little insecure about my ability to really help anyone.

RINPOCHE: Whatever our age, the extent to which we've practiced and applied these teachings will determine the degree to which we can help others, directly and by example. It's difficult to benefit others if we ask them to do something we ourselves don't do.

If we imitate other practitioners without understanding the teachings, we are acting like the yeti, who mimics human behavior. He sees farmers out in the field digging, and at night imitates them, throwing dirt around and making a big mess. He merely copies the farmers' actions without knowing their significance. There isn't much benefit in sitting with a wandering mind without intention or purpose, and like the yeti, we might only make a mess of things.

The point is not to pretend, but to actually practice the teachings. Regardless of our age, genuine practice will lead to great benefit for ourselves and others.

HELEN: I grew up with Catholic doctrine about right and wrong; for example, it's wrong to have sex with someone before you're married or to use birth control. I no longer hold to those tenets, but still have strong beliefs about right and wrong in other matters. In terms of moral discipline, how can we determine right from wrong for ourselves?

RINPOCHE: First carefully check your motivation, and then check the results of your actions. If the mind's poisons are increasing because of something you're doing, then that activity is harmful. What is right reduces attachment, aversion, and ignorance, and what is wrong increases them.

TERESA: What if the adult is helping the child build a sandcastle? How can we develop the perspective of that adult in our daily lives? Specifically, how can we develop the patience neces-sary to keep building castles of sand?

RINPOCHE: Awareness of the illusory nature of all appearances spontaneously gives rise to pervasive compassion for those who, bound by their belief in the truth of appearances, only perpetu-ate the causes of further suffering and endless dreaming. With that perspective, though our problems may seem relentless and hopeless, we will have the courage and conviction necessary to patiently persevere. Even if we can benefit only one being, we won't get discouraged and give up. Acting consistently with pure heart makes our accumulation and dedication of merit impeccable—a steadily increasing source of benefit for the sake of the dreamers.

TERESA: I'm trying to reconcile the teachings on impermanence with those on patience. For me, contemplating impermanence creates a huge sense of impatience. Considering the amount of negativity I have accumulated in the past, I feel that I'm run-ning out of time. How do I maintain patience while applying the teachings on impermanence?

RINPOCHE: If you knew that you were going to die in three hours, you wouldn't listen to anyone who told you to sit back and relax. It would be obvious that there was no time to waste. Nor would you have time to be patient if someone were drowning. You would need to jump in! We don't have time to be patient in our efforts to purify karma. What we think is patience in that case is just laziness. Tulku Arik slept only one hour a night from the time he was thirteen, practicing diligently for the rest of his life.

Where we do need to be patient is in avoiding nonvirtue, creating virtue, and nurturing bodhicitta. With that kind of patience, we can swiftly accomplish the path.

ORLIN: I appreciate the value of everything you've said, but I have to admit that it all seems a bit too much. It's hard to imagine someone like me being able to really put these teachings into practice.

RINPOCHE: I think that those of you at this peace training truly have good heart. I am not trying to force a particular spiritual path on any of you. But it is important that you recognize the gift of your life right now because you will lose it all too soon. Don't think that you lack what it takes to accomplish something of great benefit. Don't let this opportunity slip through your fingers.

Whether or not we believe in samsara, here we are. And whether or not we believe in the poisons of the mind, we still have them. If we are sick, why deny that medicine can help us? We may say that we aren't ready for the spiritual path, but death isn't going to wait until we are. We're willing to drink poison, but when it comes to taking medicine, we say that we're not ready or we don't have confidence in the diagnosis or the prescription.

If whales and dolphins can learn to dance, how can we say we can't practice patience or do spiritual practice? We have the necessary skills; we just need to apply them.

18

The Radiant Heart

TIBETANS HAVE A SAYING: At the last moment, there is nothing much to say. All the same, I have a few last thoughts to share.

The teachings we have discussed here are infallible. They are part of an ancient tradition that has consistently shown countless generations of practitioners the way to liberation. My intention in offering them is that you carry them into the world in your radiant and open hearts. Each of us is a nexus in a vast web of interdependent relationships. If we sincerely practice these teachings, everyone in our lives will benefit, and our kindness toward those close to us will gradually extend to the world at large. Though it is difficult to imagine, if we can help even one person and dedicate the merit to all beings, we will create immeasurable benefit that pervades all of time and space.

Remember always that the purpose of these teachings is to provide means of increasing outer and inner peace for all beings, now and ultimately. If we are genuine practitioners of the bodhisattva path, others will be touched by our qualities. Everyone is searching for happiness. Those around us won't miss the changes we've undergone.

We must first have something before we can hope to give it to others. If we have good heart, it will naturally radiate to those around us. It will permeate their minds and awaken their own;

in turn, they will pass it on to others. The process is very simple and direct, and begins with our own mind.

Developing bodhicitta doesn't require giving up worldly life. Rather, it is a matter of bringing love, compassion, and awareness to everything we do. Without training in the methods that transform the mind, we won't accomplish much. But if we continually work with our mind, we can attain realization.

When I was growing up in Tibet, many of my family members outwardly led ordinary lives while inwardly doing strong spiritual practice. I myself have seen four people achieve what is called rainbow body. They had purified all of their karma and obscurations, and as a result their body transformed at the time of death into one of light. These were not monks or renunciates living in caves, but seemingly regular people who worked hard and loved their families.

With consistent practice, the mind will relax, and we'll start to see through our delusion and confusion. We'll create more virtue and less harm. In this way, our ordinary life will become a spiritual path.

DAILY LIFE AS A SPIRITUAL PATH

When you wake up each morning, instead of rising mindlessly, sit for a few moments and contemplate your good fortune: "How wonderful—I've lived through the night!" Many people go to bed healthy and never wake up. Death is very simple. We breathe out and don't breathe in again.

Think to yourself, "I don't know if I have one more day or many. But I will use the time I have well. I'll work for the happiness of others in any way I can, and if I'm not able to help, at least I'll strive not to harm any being—physically, verbally, or mentally." With this resolution, focus on the direction you want the day to take. Your ability to benefit others will increase in proportion to the scope of your intention. Then invoke the blessings of your object of faith, praying that whatever you do will benefit all beings and lead you to realize your true nature.

Throughout the day, apply the four immeasurable qualities and the four thoughts to all of your activities. Every door you open can be the heart's door to greater compassion. Every meal you purely offer can nourish all beings with loving kindness. Everything you purchase can bring to mind the transitory nature of all things.

Never overlook an opportunity to create virtue. The merit of helping others, dedicated to all beings, is boundless and becomes a powerful force for positive change.

Don't burden others with your expectations. Understanding their limitations can inspire compassion instead of disappointment, ensuring beneficial and workable relationships. Remember that you have only a short time together. Be grateful for each day you share.

Try to resist responding negatively to difficult situations. Every moment of miserliness, hatred, jealousy, or pride drives you more deeply into suffering. These poisons only further obscure the crystal, your inherent perfection. Instead, cultivate acceptance and contentment.

When you feel upset or depressed, focusing on the suffering of others is genuinely helpful. Regardless of how overwhelming your circumstances may seem, those of countless others are much worse. Putting yourself in their shoes brings perspective to your own situation.

Continually contemplate impermanence. Whatever you desire, dislike, think, or feel is impermanent. Words of praise or blame are impermanent. They all come and go. With this understanding, you won't be so upset by the dramas of daily life.

Outwardly you can continue to make plans, but inwardly cultivate nonattachment. When death comes, it won't do any good to cling to plans, no matter how well-intentioned they may be. When death takes your last breath, you need to really know that everything you are leaving is impermanent—a dream—and let go.

Continue to practice contemplation and relaxation. You don't have to sit on a special cushion, in a special room, with special incense. Do it wherever you are: in line at the convenience store, driving to work, taking a shower, doing dishes. The more you practice, the more quickly your faults will diminish and your positive qualities will increase. Revealing mind's perfection is simply a matter of repetition—bringing your awareness back to one or another of these meditations again and again.

When you go to bed at night, review the day. Reflect on the virtue and negativity you created. Really check. Be honest. If you caused harm, don't become discouraged, but make a commitment to change. Using the four powers of purification, imagine that you are cleansed of all sickness, negativity, obscurations, and karmic debts, until not even the residue of your harmful actions remains. Then allow your mind to settle into the openness and compassion that are the blessings of your object of faith. Dedicate all the virtue you've ever accumulated to the temporary and ultimate happiness of all beings without exception. Then go to sleep.

PRACTICING WITHIN A SPIRITUAL TRADITION

Don't be too cautious about the spiritual path, fearful of beginning the journey. Be cautious instead about anger, greed, and ignorance. Our state of mind is like a sickness. Now is the time to take medicine, not when we're on our deathbed.

Once you've decided to begin spiritual practice, carefully determine which path works best for you. Each religion has its own complete tradition, with its own qualities. Spiritual traditions originate in response to the suffering of beings in a particular time and place. Each offers an approach that answers the needs of various kinds of people. Just as one medicine won't cure a hundred different people, the same spiritual path won't be suitable for everyone. The Buddha taught 84,000 methods for training the mind because he saw that there are 84,000 ways to be confused.

You can't assess a spiritual path adequately from the outside. It is difficult to know what it has to offer unless you actually start practicing, just as you won't know if you like something on a menu until you taste it. You can tell that a path is working for you if the poisons of your mind decrease, and loving kindness and compassion increase.

All spiritual traditions are vehicles. If you want to get somewhere, you can take a bicycle, car, train, or airplane. But if you combine the wing of a plane, the pedals of a bicycle, the steering wheel of a car, and the wheels of a train, you may arrive at your destination, or you may not. Most likely, you'll go nowhere. Worse still, your vehicle could crash, injuring yourself and others.

When you encounter a tradition that has been proven over time and continues to work for others, try it. Your life is too short to waste on a trendy, unproven path. If a tradition serves you well, follow it without distraction. There may be many well-worn paths to the mountaintop, but if we make a habit of abandoning one for another as the going gets difficult, we will merely circle the base of the mountain, never reaching our destination.

Don't criticize or judge others' paths. It is a mistake to think yours is the best or only way. Although the basic purpose of religion is to help people, attachment to yours and aversion to others' will cause divisiveness and conflict. Spiritual practice is meant to reduce the poisons of the mind, not foster them. Don't use spirituality as an excuse to indulge in pride, jealousy, greed, animosity, or harmful thinking. These are serious faults, whether we commit them in the context of spiritual or worldly life. If the medicine we take produces sickness, it is not beneficial.

We must be careful not to wear the badge of our own spiritual tradition by preaching, judging, or imposing our ideas on others. In the long run, each and every religion that teaches the value of extending kindness and refraining from harm benefits those who sincerely follow it. The great scholar Nagarjuna said that, regardless of one's tradition, faith and moral discipline will produce infallible benefit and increase mind's positive qualities. We may prefer American, Japanese, Indian, or Tibetan food, but the important thing is that we eat and are nourished, not that everyone eat the same food.

If you find yourself drawn to the Buddhist tradition, my sincere advice is that you seek out a teacher. A spiritual teacher is important because he introduces us to the causes of suffering and methods for uprooting them. But it is necessary to examine a teacher's background, lineage, and training to determine whether he is either qualified and authorized to teach or is self-appointed. Does he have a strong foundation in study and practice? Is there a difference between his words and actions? A good teacher will live the teachings, exemplifying good heart and consistently demonstrating compassion, putting his students' needs first.

If listening to and applying the teachings transforms your mind, you can be sure that the teacher-student relationship is benefiting you. Trust will arise naturally. As your mind changes, your trust will increase. As your trust grows, you will seek out more teachings, apply them, deepen your trust, and so on.

The point of our practice is not to have visionary or clair-voyant experiences, but to reduce mind's poisons and enhance our positive qualities. If that is happening, we are reducing the causes of suffering. As we apply the methods our teacher gives us, ideally we will change every day; if not, then every month, and certainly every year. Ultimately, change is the key—to change the heart, to discover mind's true nature.

I am no stranger to difficulty, but because of my training and practice, none of my experiences have been overwhelming. I know personally the power of the lama's blessings, and how beneficial contemplation and meditation can be in dealing with life's circumstances. When I was younger, whenever I received a teaching, I reviewed the material twenty-five times that same day. Now, I sometimes forget the names of my relatives, but I will never forget the teachings, because they are so firmly imprinted on my mind.

However many years I have left, I am at peace with the fact that I am going to die. Death doesn't frighten me, because I have confidence in my spiritual practice and have tried to help others as much as I can. I know from experience that these teachings will benefit anyone who applies them, not only in this life, but at the time of death and in future lives.

From the depth of my heart I tell you: one moment of kindness to another being, one act of pure intention is worth more than all the wealth in the world when you are dying. So practice now, while you can, to the greatest possible extent in every situation. This will fulfill the supreme purpose of your life, and at the time of death, you will have no regrets.

COMMITMENT

At this juncture in the Bodhisattva Peace Training, we conduct a commitment ceremony. If you wish, you can make a formal commitment to whatever you feel prepared to uphold—large or small—as a result of your participation in this training. One reason for doing this is to create a framework that will support your practice. Making and upholding commitments is also a way to accumulate merit. For example, you may be doing everything you can to love and care for your children. But from the time you make an actual commitment to doing so, you accumulate merit every moment you uphold it, and the merit you are already creating by your parenting increases. Alternatively, you could vow not to slay any dragons. I don't know if you've ever seen a dragon or if it has ever occurred to you to kill one. If you don't make such a commitment and never cross paths with a dragon, you create neither the nonvirtue of killing one nor the virtue of refraining from doing it. Nothing is at stake. Nonetheless, simply by making a commitment and keeping it, you create merit.

The commitment you make today can serve as a watershed in your life, a point of departure from who and where you were before, to who and where you want to be. Consider how you want to live your life differently, having heard, pondered, and questioned these teachings.

For the purposes of this ceremony, we make a small shrine on which we place a representation of our object of faith that symbolizes all enlightened beings, whom we invoke as witnesses to our vows. Before this representation, we make our commitments. I begin the ceremony by offering a candle that represents the lamp of wisdom I received from my teachers. As you light your own lamp from this flame, you join your intention with that of the lineage of bodhisattvas who have and always will work ceaselessly to illuminate all worlds for all beings.

From my heart, I thank you for the commitments you have made. Although you may appear as you did before, you are no longer the same. Those of you who have made commitments to harmlessness and to the temporary and ultimate benefit of others can be confident that, for you, samsaric suffering will cease. You have opened a door that you will eventually walk through.

It is important not to forget your commitments. Bring them to mind many times during the day. If you do forget or make mistakes, regret and purify them using the four powers.

DEDICATION

Each of us has made a great effort to listen to these teachings and to contemplate, ask questions, and meditate on them. Now we will dedicate the virtue of having done so, as well as all the virtue we have ever created and will create as a result of what we have learned and committed ourselves to here. Without clinging, we offer it to those with whom we have positive or negative connections, and ultimately to all who suffer in the darkness of ignorance. May the tragic causes and conditions of their suffering be fully uprooted, and may all beings attain complete realization of mind's true nature—a state of immutable, absolute, victorious peace.

~

DEDICATION PRAYER[*]

Throughout my many lives and until this moment, whatever virtue I have accomplished, including the merit generated by this practice and all that I will ever attain, this I offer for the welfare of sentient beings.

May sickness, war, famine, and suffering be decreased for every being, while their wisdom and compassion increase in this and every future life.

May I clearly perceive all experiences to be as insubstantial as the dream fabric of the night and instantly awaken to perceive the pure wisdom display in the arising of every phenomenon.

May I quickly attain enlightenment in order to work ceaselessly for the liberation of all sentient beings.

---

[*] The "Dedication Prayer" and "Prayer of Aspiration" are from the concise practice of Red Tara compiled by H.E. Chagdud Tulku Rinpoche. "The Auspicious Wish" is by Kyabjé Dudjom Rinpoche.

PRAYER OF ASPIRATION

Buddhas and bodhisattvas all together, whatever
   kind of motivation you have,
whatever kind of beneficial action,
whatever kind of wishing prayers,
whatever kind of omniscience,
whatever kind of life accomplishment,
whatever kind of benevolent power,
and whatever kind of immense wisdom you have,
then similarly I, who have come in the same way
   to benefit beings, pray to attain these qualities.

THE AUSPICIOUS WISH

At this very moment, for the peoples and the nations of the
earth, may not even the names disease, famine, war, and suffering be heard.

Rather may their moral conduct, merit, wealth, and pros-
perity increase, and may supreme good fortune and well-being
always arise for them.

HIS EMINENCE CHAGDUD TULKU RINPOCHE, a highly revered Tibetan meditation master, taught widely throughout the world and established many centers for the study and practice of Vajrayana Buddhism. His main centers are Chagdud Gonpa Rigdzin Ling in Junction City, California, and Chagdud Khadro Ling in Três Coroas, Brazil.

LAMA SHENPEN DROLMA was ordained as a lama by H.E. Chagdud Tulku Rinpoche in 1996. She is the resident lama of Iron Knot Ranch, a retreat center under development in southern New Mexico, where she is establishing the Bodhisattva Peace Institute to bring to fruition Chagdud Rinpoche's vision of making the Bodhisattva Peace Training widely available throughout the world.

Visit www.ironknot.org/bpi for more information about the Bodhisattva Peace Institute at Iron Knot Ranch.

AS WE TAKE THESE TEACHINGS to heart, may the aspiration of Chagdud Tulku Rinpoche be fulfilled: that the light of the awakened mind radiate outwards, like one candle illuminating the next, until the entire world is filled with light.

OTHER TITLES OF INTEREST FROM
IRON KNOT PRESS

Sunlight on Shadows: Embracing Great Compassion,
Lama Shenpen Drolma

OTHER TITLES OF INTEREST FROM
PADMA PUBLISHING

*Gates to Buddhist Practice: Essential Teachings of a Tibetan
Master,* Chagdud Tulku

Life in Relation to Death, Chagdud Tulku

*Lord of the Dance: The Autobiography
of a Tibetan Lama,* Chagdud Tulku

Finding Freedom: Writings from Death Row,
Jarvis Jay Masters

www.ingramcontent.com/pod-product-compliance
Lightning Source LLC
Chambersburg PA
CBHW031125090426
42738CB00008B/979